Techniques for Peripheral Interventions

Dierk Scheinert, Andrej Schmidt, Giancarlo Biamino

Techniques for Peripheral Interventions

Interactive DVD included

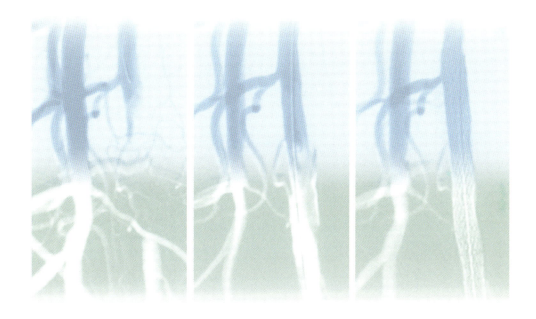

In collaboration with

Piergiorgio Cao

Horst Sievert

URBAN & VOGEL

Dierk Scheinert, MD
Andrej Schmidt, MD
Giancarlo Biamino, MD

University of Leipzig - Heart Center
Department of Clinical and
Interventional Angiology
Parkkrankenhaus Leipzig Südost GmbH
Department of Internal Medicine I -
Angiology and Cardiology
Strümpellstraße 39-41
04289 Leipzig, Germany

Under an unrestricted educational grant from Invatec.

Bibliographic information published by Die Deutsche Bibliothek
Die Deutsche Bibliothek lists this publication in the Deutsche Nationalbibliografie; detailed bibliographic data are available in the Internet at http://dnb.ddb.de.

The use of registered names, trademarks, etc. in this publication does not imply, even in the absence of a specific statement, that such names are exempt from the relevant protective laws and regulations and therefore free for general use.
Product liability: The publisher can give no guarantee for information about drug dosage and application thereof contained in this book. In every individual case the respective user must check its accuracy by consulting other pharmaceutical literature.

All rights reserved
© Urban & Vogel GmbH, Munich 2007
Urban & Vogel is a publishing company of Springer Science+Business Media GmbH

Composition: Atelier59, Munich
Printing and binding:
fgb. freiburger graphische betriebe, www.fgb.de
Printed in Germany

ISBN 13: 978-3-89935-190-3
ISBN 10: 3-89935-190-8

Contents DVD

***Iliac Arteries** (Chapter 2)*
- Stent-supported reconstruction of the aortic bifurcation (1)
- Reconstruction of the aortic bifurcation with kissing stents (2)*
- Recanalization of a right common iliac artery occlusion (3)
- Recanalization of a right external iliac artery occlusion (4)

***Femoropopliteal Arteries** (Chapter 3)*
- PTA of SFA stenoses (5)
- Laser recanalization of a right SFA occlusion (6)*
- Endovascular atherectomy for SFA in-stent restenosis (7)*
- Subintimal recanalization with the Pioneer catheter (8)*

***Infrapopliteal Arteries** (Chapter 4)*
- PTA of the anterior tibial artery for CLI (9)
- Multilevel recanalization of left SFA and ATA (10)

***Renal Arteries** (Chapter 5)*
- PTA and stenting of left renal artery (11)

***Thoracic Aorta** (Chapter 6)*
- Endovascular repair of a descending thoracic aortic aneurysm (12)*
- Stent-graft implantation for type B aortic dissection (13)*

***Abdominal Aorta** (Chapter 7)*
- Endovascular repair of an abdominal aortic aneurysm (14)

***Supraaortic Arteries** (Chapter 8)*
- Recanalization of left subclavian artery occlusion (15)
- Carotid artery stenting with filter protection (16)
- Carotid artery stenting with proximal protection (17)

*Images from Euro PCR 2003 under the authorisation of Europa Organisation

Contents

	Preface	7
Chapter One	Clinical Evaluation and Vascular Laboratory Testing for Peripheral Arterial Occlusive Disease	8
Chapter Two	Recanalization of the Pelvic Arteries	26
Chapter Three	Recanalization of the Femoropopliteal Tract	44
Chapter Four	Below-the-Knee Interventions	70
Chapter Five	Endovascular Intervention of Renal Artery Stenosis	94
Chapter Six	Endovascular Therapy of Aneurysms and Dissections of the Thoracic Aorta	110
Chapter Seven	Endoluminal Treatment of Abdominal Aortic Aneurysm	124
Chapter Eight	Carotid Stenting: Technical Aspects and Clinical Results	142
	Index	174

Preface

In the field of peripheral vascular disease, knowledge and technology continue to advance rapidly. Nevertheless, the endovascular approach to the treatment of obstructive lesions, particularly in the femoropopliteal tract, continues to be object of controversial discussion.

In concomitance with these facts, there have been relevant "philosophic changes" in the management of sclerotic, obstructive vascular disease.

On the one hand, the lack of evidence-based long-term results of controlled studies fuels the dispute; on the other hand, the recent published results using advanced technologies and, in particular, new generations of dedicated peripheral stents indicate a potential breakthrough in the successful treatment also of long occlusions and complex multilevel obstructions.

The goal of this book is to cover the different technical aspects regarding the endovascular treatment of arterial disease in the different regions of interest. We tried to maintain the text clinically oriented, and we hope that it can be considered a practical guide particularly for interventionalists starting the peripheral program.

Because of the relatively small amount of evidence-based data, many aspects presented in the different chapters are derived from our daily practice and reflect nearly two decades of personal experience in the endovascular field.

For this reason, the book and the related DVD contain a large number of examples showing our day-to-day practice and offering a broad range of techniques and case material. The presented cases are ment to illustrate indications, strategic decision points, as well as equipment selection. We intentionally limited the presentation of premature – not clinically extensively tested – technologies in the continuously evolving field of endovascular treatment.

Readers are invited to contribute to the success of this book by expressing their constructive criticism.

Leipzig, August 2006

Prof. Giancarlo Biamino
on behalf of the authors

Chapter One

Clinical Evaluation and Vascular Laboratory Testing for Peripheral Arterial Occlusive Disease

Introduction

Peripheral arterial occlusive disease (PAOD) is a common and often underdiagnosed manifestation of atherosclerosis. The rapidly evolving possibilities of endovascular revascularization for many arterial regions make screening and accurate noninvasive diagnostic evaluation more and more important.

A complete history and physical examination is the essential first step in evaluating patients for a possible endovascular intervention. For the diagnosis of PAOD of the lower extremities, several qualitative and quantitative noninvasive tests are useful, like Doppler ultrasonography, pulse volume recording, segmental blood pressure measurement, exercise testing, transcutaneous oxymetry, and color-coded duplex sonography. Each test has its specific utility and can be used either individually or in combination with other noninvasive tests to obtain information about the hemodynamic and functional severity of peripheral atherosclerosis in patients with claudication.

The present chapter attempts to give recommendations for a practical noninvasive workup of the patient with PAOD.

Lower Limb Arterial Disease

Clinical Evaluation

Intermittent claudication is the most common symptom in PAOD of the lower limbs. The patient feels pain or tightness, sometimes only tiredness or numbness of the extremity during exercise. On the basis of the clinical history, it is almost always possible to distinguish between vascular intermittent claudication and pseudoclaudication due to nonvascular causes. Vascular claudication is usually strongly exercise-dependent, and relief of symptoms occurs only after minutes of rest. The part of the limb involved lies usually one level distal to the diseased arterial segment.

PAOD is classified using the Fontaine staging system or Rutherford classification *(Table 1)*. The anamnesis should report the initial walking capacity, the distance at which the patient first experiences claudication with exertion, and the absolute walking capacity, which is the distance when the patient can no longer ambulate. With advancing disease or acute ischemia,

TABLE 1

Clinical categories of peripheral arterial occlusive disease. The Fontaine and Rutherford classifications.
AP: ankle pressure;
BP: blood pressure;
PVR: pulse volume reading.

TABLE 1.

Fontaine	Clinical description	Rutherford	Clinical description	Objective criteria
I	Asymptomatic	0	Asymptomatic	Normal exercise test
IIa	Mild claudication, walks > 200 m on standardized treadmill test	1	Mild claudication	Completes exercise test, AP after exercise < 50 mmHg but > 25 mmHg less than BP
IIb	Moderate to severe claudication, walks < 200 m on standardized treadmill test	2	Moderate claudication	Between category 1 and 3
		3	Severe claudication	Cannot complete exercise test and AP after exercise < 50 mmHg
III	Ischemic rest pain	4	Ischemic rest pain	Resting AP < 40 mmHg, flat or barely pulsatile ankle PVR, toe pressure < 30 mmHg
IV	Ulceration or gangrene	5	Minor tissue loss – non-healing ulcers, focal gangrene with diffuse pedal edema	Resting AP < 60 mmHg, flat or barely pulsatile ankle PVR, toe pressure < 40 mmHg
		6	Major tissue loss – extending above metatarsal level	Same as category 5

patients may complain of a sudden decrease in the initial claudication distance, disabling claudication, or rest pain. If critical ischemia is not treated aggressively, progression to ischemic ulceration, gangrene, loss of motor and/or sensory function and, eventually, limb loss can occur. In diabetic patients, critical ischemia with ulcerations or gangrene may be present without warning signs like deterioration of the walking capacity or rest pain.

Physical findings that support the diagnosis of PAOD of the lower limb include decreased skin temperature, shiny, hairless skin over the lower extremities, dystrophic toenails, pallor on elevation of the extremity, and rubor when the limb is dependent. Further examination may reveal bruits over the abdominal aorta, iliac or femoral arteries, and absent or decreased peripheral pulses. An attempt to rule out an abdominal aortic aneurysm should always be carried out.

The Ankle-Brachial Index

The Ankle-Brachial Index (ABI) measurement is one of the most reproducible and easily to conduct tests to objectively define the severity of limb ischemia. The tools required to obtain an ABI include a blood pressure cuff and a continuous wave (cw) Doppler probe. Blood pressure is measured in both upper extremities, and the highest systolic reading is recorded. The ankle systolic pressure is similarly measured, using the blood pressure cuff over the distal calf and a hand-held Doppler probe examining the dorsalis pedis or posterior tibial artery. The ABI is calculated by dividing the ankle pressure (the higher of the posterior tibial or dorsalis pedis artery pressure) by the brachial systolic pressure (the higher of the two arm pressures). An ABI of ≥ 0.9 is considered to be normal, an index of 0.89–0.41 is found in mild to moderate PAOD, corresponding classifications are Rutherford's category 2–3 or Fontaine's stage II. An ABI ≤ 0.4 or an ankle pressure < 40–50 mmHg indicates severe lower extremity arterial disease (*Table 2*).

Some limitations apply to the ABI. In patients with severe medial calcification, like in high age, diabetes mellitus and end-stage renal disease, it might be impossible to compress the arteries of the calf by the blood pressure cuff. This can result in highly elevated ankle pressures, often > 220 mmHg, leading to a falsely normal ABI. In these cases, the ABI cannot be used for diagnostic workup.

Other noninvasive tests like pulse curve recording or thorough duplex scanning will sufficiently help to evaluate the PAOD in these patients.

Another situation, where the ABI is not reliable, is the patient with distal abdominal aortic or common iliac artery

TABLE 2.

ABI	Severity of PAOD
≥ 0.9	Normal
0.7–0.89	Mild
0.41–0.69	Moderate
≤ 0.4	Severe

TABLE 2 *Relationship between Ankle-Brachial Index (ABI) and clinical severity of peripheral arterial occlusive disease (PAOD).*

TIPS AND TRICKS

- *The ABI can be misleading in diabetic patients.*

stenosis or occlusion. In these patients the ABI at rest may be normal, and measurement of the ABI after exercise is the method of choice.

Exercise Testing

Determination of both the pain-free or initial and the maximum or absolute walking distances is part of a routine workup of PAOD patients. With a constant speed of 2 miles per hour, the walking capacity is measured either with a fixed incline of 12% for up to 5 min, or with a variable incline starting at 0% with an increase of 3.5% every 2–3 min up to a maximum incline of 18%. Treadmill testing with measurement of the ABI after exercise is extremely helpful in patients with unclear symptoms and normal ABI at rest. The alterations of interest after exercise are the immediate decrease of the ankle systolic pressure and the time of recovery to the initial resting value.

A normal response to exercise can be a slight increase of the pressure but also a slight decrease of not more than 10% of the ankle systolic pressure at rest. The test is clearly positive, if the ankle pressure decreases by at least 20 mmHg, reaching the initial value only after a 5-min time interval.

The measurement of ankle pressure after exercise is useful in the demonstration of the significance of lesions, which appear as moderate stenoses on angiography, stenoses of the aortoiliac region, and for differentiation of the causes of symptoms in patients who may have pseudoclaudication associated with neurospinal disorders, especially when arterial disease coexists.

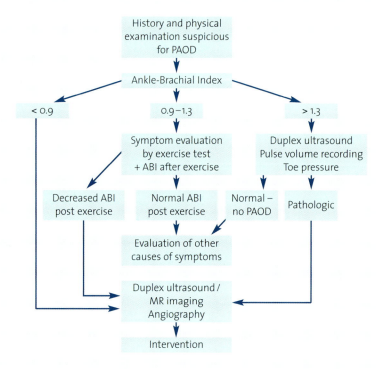

FIGURE 1. *Algorithm for the evaluation of peripheral arterial occlusive disease (PAOD).*
ABI: Ankle-Brachial Index; MR: magnetic resonance.

> **TIPS AND TRICKS**
>
> ■ *ABI measurement after exercise is a very important tool in suspected PAOD.*

However, measurement of the ABI after stress does not add practical information if it is already clearly abnormal at rest. In patients with intermittent claudication, the ABI does not necessarily predict the walking distance. The decision for therapy should be made with regard to the impairment of quality of life rather than Doppler pressure values or other diagnostic tools (Figure 1).

Duplex Scanning for the Evaluation of Lower Limb Arterial Disease

Although diagnosis can usually be made on the basis of a thorough history and physical examination in combination with a treadmill test and measurement of the ankle pressure, duplex scanning fulfills an important role in clinical practice. Especially in superficial vascular segments like the common femoral artery (CFA), the deep femoral artery, the superficial femoral artery (SFA) above the adductor canal and the popliteal artery, image quality of duplex ultrasound is excellent. Deeper located vessels such as the abdominal aorta, the pelvic arteries, the SFA at the level of the adductor canal, and parts of the lower leg arteries are less accessible by direct color-coded Doppler sonography. However, many pathologic changes can be diagnosed indirectly by changes in the spectral waveform distal to the lesion.

Pelvic Arteries

Scanning should begin by imaging the infrarenal aorta with a 2- to 3-MHz transducer to document any signs of aneurysmal or occlusive disease. The proximal part of the common iliac artery and the distal part of the external iliac artery can be visualized in about 80% and > 90%, respectively. The middle part of the pelvic axis can sufficiently be examined by duplex ultrasound only in about 25%, depending greatly on the adipose state and patient preparation. However, the presence of a well-palpable femoral pulse or normal Doppler signal of the CFA reliably excludes significant iliac stenosis. Normally, the Doppler waveform of the external iliac and common femoral artery has a triphasic configuration and peak flow velocity is in the range of 100–140 cm/s. Conversely, if the Doppler waveform becomes bi- or monophasic, with reduction of peak systolic and increase in end-diastolic velocity, the presence of a proximal, pressure-reducing stenosis is very likely (Figure 2).

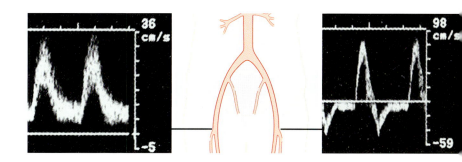

FIGURE 2. *Doppler waveform of the left common femoral artery shows a normal, triphasic morphology indicating pelvic arteries without high-grade stenosis or occlusion. Doppler sign of the right common femoral artery has a monophasic shape, found with high-grade stenosis or occlusion of the pelvic axis.*

TIPS AND TRICKS

If symptoms are suspicious for pelvic stenosis and Doppler signals of the CFA are normal, perform a treadmill test with measurement of the ABI after exercise.

> **TIPS AND TRICKS**
>
> ■ Especially in multilevel disease of the SFA also other Doppler criteria except the peak systolic velocity are used for exact quantification of the stenoses.

Femoral Arteries

Due to the superficial course of the femoropopliteal artery, the color-coded duplex sonography permits rapid location of sites of stenosis or occlusion. Using the pulsed wave (pw) Doppler a stenosis exceeding 70% can easily be diagnosed if the peak systolic velocity shows an increase of 100% with respect to the arterial segment proximal to the stenosis *(Table 3)*.

Multisegmental disease, especially of the SFA, may affect the accuracy of duplex scanning. A reduced flow distal to occluded or highly stenotic segments increases the difficulty of detecting significant Doppler velocity changes in secondary stenoses. This situation demonstrates, that the peak systolic velocity should be considered semiquantitative. Other additional duplex-sonographic parameters are very helpful in these situations. Modification of the Doppler signal from a triphasic to a bi- or monophasic waveform and various signs of turbulences indicate different degrees of the occlusive disease *(Table 3, Figure 3)*. The examination of the popliteal artery can easily give an assessment of the patency of the SFA in summary. A Doppler waveform with monophasic morphology indicates a total or functional occlusion of the vessel upstream *(Figure 4)*.

Table 3.

Grade of stenosis	Doppler waveform characteristics	PSV (cm/s)
No stenosis	Triphasic signal with minimum spectral broadening	Normal
≤ 20%	Normal waveform contour, spectral broadening	Normal
21–50%	PSV increased by 50–100% from the site proximal to the stenosis, marked spectral broadening	> 250
51–79%	Marked spectral broadening and poststenotic turbulent flow	250–350
80–90%	Marked poststenotic turbulence	> 350
Occlusion	Decreased velocities proximal and monophasic waveforms distal to the stenosis	No flow

Table 3. Duplex-sonographic criteria for semiquantitative evaluation of lower extremity artery stenoses. PSV: peak systolic velocity.

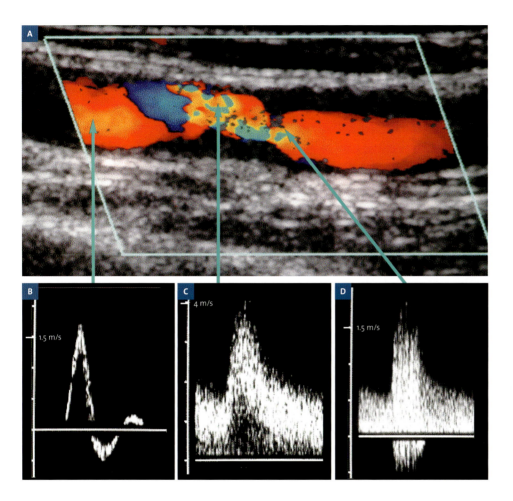

Figure 3. High-grade stenosis of the superficial femoral artery with pre-, intra- and poststenotic Doppler waveforms.
PSV: peak systolic velocity.
a) Stenosis of the superficial femoral artery.
b) Normal triphasic Doppler signal.
c) Marked spectral broadening and increase of PSV.
d) Marked spectral broadening and poststenotic turbulence.

The proximal part of the deep femoral artery should always be examined by color Doppler ultrasound. Even with angulated views, stenoses of this part of the vessel can be missed by arteriography. Duplex ultrasound gives accurate results in this region, but in concomitant stenosis or occlusion of the SFA, flow velocity may be increased in the deep femoral artery, leading to overestimation of stenosis.

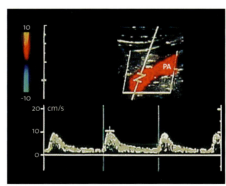

Figure 4. Monophasic Doppler waveform of the popliteal artery (PA) in a patient with an occlusion of the superficial femoral artery.

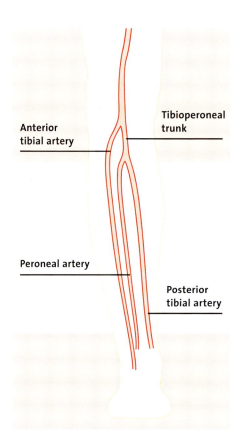

FIGURE 5.

Visibility of different infrapopliteal artery segments by duplex ultrasound.

■ *Analysis by duplex ultrasound feasible in nearly all cases.*

Analysis by duplex ultrasound not always feasible.

Infrageniculate Arteries

Studies investigating the accuracy of duplex sonography for assessment of the infrapopliteal arteries are not as uniform. A sensitivity of 59–96% and a specificity of 69–93% compared to angiography are reported for the infrageniculate region. Often, only the proximal and very distal part of the infrageniculate arteries are directly visible by duplex ultrasound *(Figure 5)*. Digital plethysmography is a very good substitution for diagnosis of arterial lesions and follow-up after angioplasty in the infrapopliteal region.

Cerebrovascular Occlusive Disease

Stroke is one of the leading causes of death in industrialized countries. Carotid artery occlusive disease is estimated to be the primary cause in up to 30% of all strokes. A complete history and physical examination, including a thorough neurologic examination to rule out the patients with neurologic symptoms referable to other causes, is the essential first step in the evaluation before a possible carotid intervention.

The most important screening method for assessing extracranial carotid, vertebral and subclavian artery disease is color-coded duplex sonography. The predominant extracranial distribution of the stenotic lesions makes them accessible to direct detection by ultrasound imaging, but also if lesions are not visible directly, the determination of indirect changes of blood flow patterns by Doppler sonography allows the correct diagnosis in the majority of cases.

Sonographic examination of the extracranial carotid arteries should be recommended not only in symptomatic patients or suspected carotid stenosis, but should be part of a complete checkup in each patient with known or suspected arteriosclerotic disease or even in case of arteriosclerotic risk factors.

Duplex Sonography for the Evaluation of Supraaortic Arteries

Internal Carotid Artery

Conventional angiography is considered to be the gold standard for evaluating the degree of carotid artery stenosis. However, this technique is invasive and not free of complications. Carotid arteries are optimal vessels for application of duplex ultrasound, providing both morphologic and hemodynamic data by combining different acquisition modalities.

In contrast to the enormous number of publications concerning the quantification of carotid stenosis, there are still uncertainties about the most precise method of measurement. Planimetry of stenosis is still in practice, however, due to the widening of the carotid bulb and proximal part of the internal carotid artery, this technique often leads to an overestimation of the stenosis.

Main signs of color Doppler used for diagnosing arterial stenoses include narrowing of the vessel lumen, the aliasing phenomenon caused by an increase of flow velocity in the stenosis, and other color phenomena like poststenotic turbulences, flow separation, and flow reversal. The main value of color Doppler is to detect the stenosed vessel segment and offer a rough estimation of the extent of luminal constriction, which then has to be examined by pw or cw Doppler technique .

Cw Doppler ultrasound is widely used for stenosis estimation. With a 4-MHz Doppler probe, a Doppler shift < 5,000 Hz indicates mild stenosis and a Doppler shift > 9,000 Hz reliably indicates high-grade stenosis *(Table 4)*.

Since with the use of cw Doppler sonography no angle correction can be performed, the Doppler parameter most widely used at present is the intrastenotic peak systolic velocity, measured by pw Doppler *(Figure 6)*. But recommended cutoff values for detection of stenoses > 70% vary widely between 1.25 m/s and 3.25 m/s, reflecting its semiquantitative character.

The ratio of internal to common carotid artery peak velocity was proposed for compensation of interindividual and interequipment variability with a value of 3 indicating a stenosis > 70% with a sensitivity of > 90% and specificity of 80%. However, because in high-grade stenosis flow velocities are reduced in the common carotid artery with wide variation, this vessel might not be an ideal reference segment for normal flow velocity. Probably the best parameter in correlating Doppler parameters with angiographic morphology is the mean velocity ratio, the relation of intrastenotic to poststenotic mean velocity *(Figure 7)*. According to the principle of continuity of flow in the unbranching internal carotid artery, this method is the only one, which can compensate for interindividual and interequipment variability simultaneously. If the examiner is not yet used to this method, it might be difficult in the beginning to obtain velocity data in the distal internal carotid artery of patients with high carotid bifurcations. The poststenotic velocity has to be measured 4–5 cm distal to the stenosis, where

TIPS AND TRICKS

■ *The peak systolic velocity within the stenosis is a semiquantitative measurement and can be misleading for example in contralateral occlusion.*

FIGURE 6. *Criteria for semiquantitative estimation of the degree of internal carotid artery stenoses. ICA/CCA: internal carotid artery/common carotid artery.*

TABLE 4.

Degree of stenosis	≤ 50%	60%	70%	80%	90%	95%
Continuous wave Doppler shift (kHz)	< 4	4	7	10	> 10	Variable
Systolic max. pulsed wave Doppler velocity (cm/s)	< 120	120	200	300	> 300	Variable
End-diastolic pulsed wave Doppler velocity (cm/s)	< 130			> 130		Variable
ICA/CCA Index	< 1.5	≥ 1.5	≥ 2	≥ 4	> 5	

blood flow without turbulence is re-established *(Figure 8)*. Using sensitive color Doppler systems and suitable curved array or sector probes, < 5% of all patients will be found ineligible for distal velocity ratio measurements. A mean velocity ratio of > 5 was found to be the most accurate parameter indicating a stenosis > 70% with a sensitivity of 97% and a specificity of 98%. Irrespective of the method used for assessment of carotid stenosis, it is still recommended to vascular laboratories to validate their duplex criteria against angiographic ones. Finally, crucial for an exact assessment of carotid stenosis is the experience of the sonographer, who will often use a combination of different Doppler- und duplex-sonographic parameters.

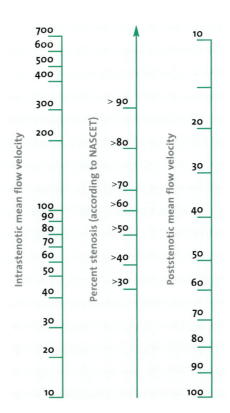

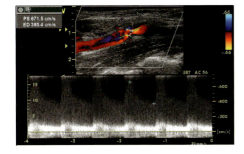

Figure 6. *High-grade stenosis of the internal carotid artery with a peak systolic velocity of >600 cm/s indicating an approximately 90% stenosis.*

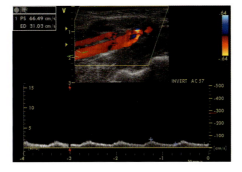

Figure 8. *Measurement of the poststenotic velocity in the same patient as in Figure 6.*

Figure 7. *Nomogram for determination of the percentage of stenosis of the internal carotid artery following the continuity equation (mean flow velocity in the stenosis in relationship to mean flow velocity behind the stenosis). The degree of stenosis corresponds to the percentage of stenosis, as it is defined by the angiographic criteria used in the North American Symptomatic Carotid Endarterectomy Trial (NASCET).*

Subclavian Artery

Duplex examination of the subclavian artery is indicated in symptomatic patients suffering from dyspraxia intermittens or paresis of the arm or embolic digital ischemia, and also includes patients with signs of vertebrobasilar insufficiency like vertigo and dizziness, syncope, or other neurologic deficits during arm exercise or arm elevation. Finally, in patients with a left internal mammary artery bypass and a coronary steal syndrome, a thorough examination of the subclavian artery is required.

Visualization of the subclavian artery by duplex ultrasound is possible in nearly all cases at least for the distal part of the vessel. Unfortunately, stenoses and occlusions mainly occur at the origin of the artery. The proximal part of the right subclavian artery as well as the distal part of the innominate artery are visible in most cases, but the origin of the left subclavian artery, where the incidence of lesions is three times higher compared to the right side, is hardly ever directly visible by duplex ultrasound. Since stenoses or occlusions are most often located proximal to the origin of the vertebral arteries, a subclavian steal phenomenon occurs, which is easily diagnosed by duplex ultrasound through demonstration of a retrograde flow in the vertebral artery of the affected side and substantiated by poststenotic or postocclusive Doppler spectra recorded in the distal subclavian artery. If the subclavian stenosis is of moderate degree, only minor alterations might be detected in the ipsilateral vertebral artery like an attenuated systolic flow ("systolic deceleration") or an alternating flow *(Figure 9, Figure 10a)*. In this case, provocative tests can verify the diagnosis of a stress-induced subclavian steal syndrome *(Figure 10b)*. For example, after release of a pressure cuff stopping the arterial blood flow at the level of the brachial artery, the oxygen demand of the arm will lead to an increased blood flow in the vertebral and brachial arteries, which will turn the duplex-sonographic alternating Doppler sign of the vertebral artery into a complete retrograde Doppler waveform. In case of a high-grade stenosis or occlusion of the subclavian artery, the retrograde flow of the vertebral artery will be amplified for several minutes, which might be combined with dizziness or vertigo.

Color-coded duplex sonography is the method of choice to verify subclavian artery stenoses or occlusions and subclavian steal phenomenon with an overall accuracy of > 95%. Further examinations by digital subtraction angiography (DSA) or magnetic resonance angiography (MRA) are only necessary in symptomatic patients before intervention.

> **TIPS AND TRICKS**
>
> ■ *Quantification of subclavian artery stenoses is based on duplex-sonographic examination of both vertebral and both subclavian arteries.*

Preinterventional Diagnosis

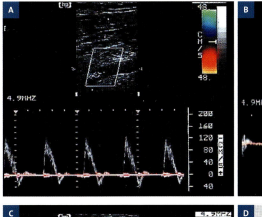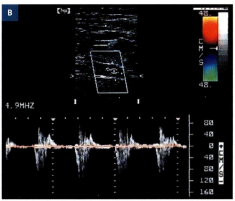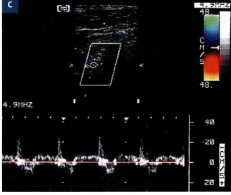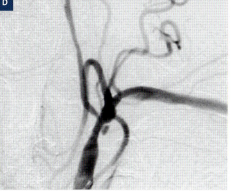

FIGURES 9A TO 9D.

a) Doppler waveform of the unstenosed right subclavian artery.
b) Doppler waveform visualizing poststenotic turbulences in the left subclavian artery.
c) Doppler waveform of the left vertebral artery showing an orthograde flow during systole and a retrograde flow during diastole corresponding to an incomplete subclavian steal phenomenon.
d) Angiography of the left subclavian artery indicating a 50–60% stenosis in the same patient.

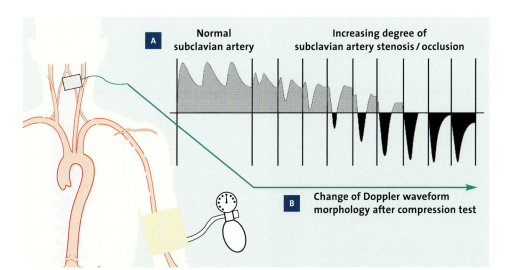

FIGURES 10A AND 10B.

a) Doppler waveform of the vertebral artery in dependence of the degree of stenosis of the prevertebral subclavian artery.
b) Change of Doppler waveform of the vertebral artery after release of a suprasystolic compression of the arm of 3–5 min duration.

Renal Artery Stenosis

Screening for renal artery stenosis (RAS) is indicated in patients with suspected renovascular hypertension or ischemic nephropathy. The critical requirements for a clinically useful screening test include safety, low cost, and a high sensitivity or a low false-negative rate. Arteriography remains the gold standard for the diagnosis of renal artery disease, but it is unsuitable for screening because of its high cost and invasive nature.

Several Doppler criteria have been developed for duplex ultrasound diagnosis of RAS. These include intrastenotic peak systolic velocity (*Figure 11*), ratio of renal intrastenotic to aortic peak systolic velocity, broadening of the Doppler spectra, and ratio of the peak systolic to end-diastolic velocities. An intrastenotic peak systolic velocity of 180–200 cm/s and a renal to aortic peak systolic ratio of at least 3.0–3.5 are generally accepted as cutoff for a relevant RAS. These parameters depend on the identification of hemodynamic changes that occur directly at the site of the arterial stenosis, which necessitates duplex scanning of the renal arteries by a transabdominal approach. In practice, however, in a considerable percentage of patients the ostium of the renal artery is not sufficiently visible despite the use of color Doppler sonography. Another limitation of renal duplex scanning is the failure in identifying accessory renal arteries, which have an incidence of 25%. Furthermore, even if renal arteries are successfully visualized, it may be difficult to determine the exact course, so that angle-corrected velocity determinations are often inaccurate. To overcome these limitations associated with direct scanning of the renal arteries, a different, indirect approach by evaluation of intrarenal arterial Doppler waveforms can be chosen. With the lateral approach to the kidney and with guidance of color Doppler flow imaging, Doppler examination of intrarenal arteries is easier to perform and rates of inadequate or

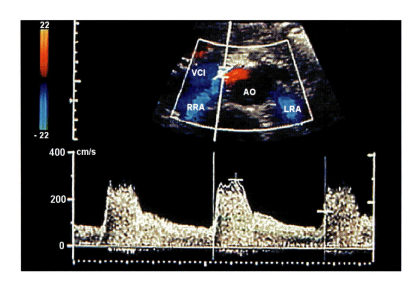

Figure 11. *High-grade stenosis of the right renal artery (RRA). AO: aorta; LRA: left renal artery; VCI: vena cava inferior.*

incomplete examinations are much lower. In addition, from a pathophysiologic point of view, Doppler flow analysis at the level of parenchymal arteries might more clearly reflect the pressure gradient to which the afferent arteriolar baroreceptor of the juxtaglomerular region is subjected and, thus, may be more reliable in determining the hemodynamic importance of RAS *(Figure 12)*.

For diagnosis of a relevant stenosis of > 75%, an acceleration time of the systolic rise of > 80 ms and an acceleration of < 1 m/s² are accepted to have a high sensitivity and specificity. However, the most common parameter is the Pourcelot or Resistive Index (RI), which is calculated using the following equation *(Figure 13)*:

[1 − (end-diastolic velocity/peak systolic velocity)]

Normal values range between 0.5 and 0.7. Parenchymal Doppler waveform and therefore renal RI, however, are influenced not only by hemodynamically relevant RAS, but also by vascular intrarenal impedance, with high values related to high impedance. Alterations in arteriolar tone, for example due to vasoactive drugs or microangiopathy as well as to acute and chronic renal disease, potentially have an effect on the Doppler waveform. In addition, various other factors like patient age, heart rate, blood pressure, aortic valve disease, and others are known to affect renal RI. Calculation of ΔRI by use of the contralateral mean renal RI as an intraindividual standard eliminates the effects of various factors mentioned above. It is believed, that ΔRI permits much more sensitive identification of substantial RAS as well as discrimination between moderate and severe stenosis than RI. A ΔRI of 5% has proven to be a sufficient predictor of hemodynamically relevant stenosis. An important limitation though, is the occurrence of bilateral renal arterial stenosis.

Renal Doppler sonography has been studied over the last 15 years for its potential as a first-line diagnostic test for RAS. The results of these studies have been different and sometimes inconsistent. With the use of single Doppler parameter or various combinations of criteria, sensitivity was found to be 75–96% and specificity 62–100%. By contrast, some prospective studies have shown sensitivities as low as 0% and specificities down to 37% due to a high percentage of insufficient visibility of

> **TIPS AND TRICKS**
>
> ■ Duplex sonography of the renal arteries includes examination of the origin of the artery and measurement of the Resistive Index (RI) of at least three segmental arteries of both kidneys.

FIGURES 12A AND 12B.
a) Normal Doppler signal of the segmental renal arteries with a normal Resistive Index of 0.68.
b) Doppler signal of segmental arteries in high-grade stenosis of the main renal artery, Resistive Index of 0.45.

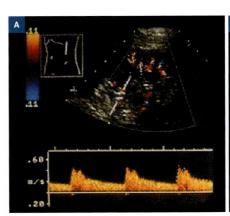
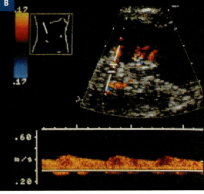

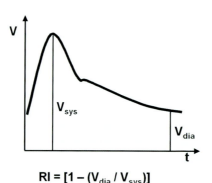

FIGURE 13. *Determination of the Pourcelot or Resistive Index (RI).*

Summary

the proximal part of the renal arteries. However, these contradictory results most probably reflect the challenging character of this examination.

Renal duplex scanning may also provide a method for predicting the clinical outcome of renal revascularization. Radermacher et al. found, that a renal RI of at least 0.8 before revascularization is a strong predictor of worsening renal function and lack of improvement in blood pressure despite the correction of RAS. Conversely, lower RI values are associated with an improvement in both renal function and blood pressure after the correction of RAS. This preinterventional test might have important potentials to reduce postinterventional failures, if ongoing studies will confirm these findings.

In PAOD of the lower limb, clinical history and physical examination are reliable for making the diagnosis. Several noninvasive tests are available to confirm the suspected diagnosis, and of these, determination of the ABI and the exercise treadmill test are most important. Duplex sonography provides accurate information on specific areas of stenosis and can replace routine preinterventional angiography in a substantial number of patients. Duplex scanning also has become the primary diagnostic method for follow-up of patients after interventional or surgical procedures of the lower limb.

Furthermore, color-coded duplex and Doppler ultrasonography is the most important method in the evaluation of supraaortic arteries. Its accuracy in calculating the degree of internal carotid stenosis matches that of the "gold standard" angiography. It is the first-choice diagnostic test in suspected subclavian artery disease as well.

Currently, duplex scanning in a qualified vascular laboratory represents the best screening test for renal artery stenosis.

It should also be the first noninvasive technique applied for the detection of peripheral aneurysms, pseudoaneurysms, arteriovenous fistulae, and assessment of arteriopathy of many other regions not mentioned in this article.

References

1. Allard L, Cloutier G, Guo Z, Durand LG. Review of the assessment of single level and multilevel arterial occlusive disease in lower limbs by duplex ultrasound. Ultrasound Med Biol 1999;25:495–502.
2. Arbeille P, Bouin-Pineau MH, Herault S. Accuracy of the main Doppler methods for evaluating the degree of carotid stenoses (continuous wave, pulsed wave, and colour Doppler). Ultrasound Med Biol 1999;25:65–73.
3. Carpenter JP, Lexa FJ, Davis JT. Determination of duplex Doppler ultrasound criteria appropriate to the North American Symptomatic Carotid Endarterectomy Trial. Stroke 1996;27:695–9.
4. Creager MA. Clinical assessment of the patient with claudication: the role of the vascular laboratory. Vasc Med 1997;2:231–7.
5. House MK, Dowling RJ, King P, Gibson RN. Using Doppler sonography to reveal renal artery stenosis: an evaluation of optimal imaging parameters. AJR Am J Roentgenol 1999;173:761–5.
6. Hua HT, Hood DB, Jensen CC, Hanks SE, Weaver FA. The use of colour flow duplex scanning to detect significant renal artery stenosis. Ann Vasc Surg 2000;14:118–24.
7. Koelemay MJW, den Hartog D, Prins MH, Kromhout JG, Legemate DA, Jacobs MJ. Diagnosis of arterial disease of the lower extremities with duplex ultrasonography. Br J Surg 1996;83:404–9.
8. Landwehr P, Schulte O, Voshage G. Ultrasound examination of carotid and vertebral arteries. Eur Radiol 2001;11:1521–34.
9. Motew SJ, Cherr GS, Craven TE, Travis JA, Wong JM, Reavis SW, Hansen KJ. Renal duplex sonography: main renal artery versus hilar analysis. J Vasc Surg 2000;32: 462–9, 469–71.
10. North American Symptomatic Carotid Endarterectomy Trial. Methods, patient characteristics, and progress. Stroke 1991;22:711–20.
11. Pemberton M, London NJ. Colour flow duplex imaging of occlusive arterial disease of the lower limb. Br J Surg 1997;84:912–9.
12. Radermacher J, Chavan A, Bleck J, Vitzthum A, Stoess B, Gebel MJ, Galinski M, Koch KM, Haller H. Use of Doppler ultrasonography to predict the outcome of therapy for renal-artery stenosis. N Engl J Med 2001; 344:410–7.
13. Ranke C, Creutzig A, Becker H, Trappe HJ. Standardization of carotid ultrasound: a hemodynamic method to normalize for interindividual and interequipment variability. Stroke 1999;30:402–6.
14. Rutherford RB, Baker JD, Ernst C, Johnston KW, Porter JM, Ahn S, Jones DN. Recommended standards for reports dealing with lower extremity ischemia: revised version. J Vasc Surg 1997;26:517–38.

Chapter Two

Recanalization of the Pelvic Arteries

Introduction

About one third of the obstructive lesions in peripheral arterial occlusive disease (PAOD) affect the aortoiliac segment. Iliac artery obstructions have traditionally been treated with aortofemoral or aorto-bifemoral graft surgery. Although highly effective, these surgical interventions are associated with a substantial procedure-related risk for the patient. In a meta-analysis of data published after 1975, the aggregate operative mortality rate was 3.3%, and the aggregate systemic morbidity rate 8.3%.

Percutaneous transluminal angioplasty (PTA) is a less invasive treatment alternative, and it has proven to be an effective technique for the treatment of focal iliac artery stenoses. The procedural technical success rate has improved significantly (up to 95%), especially using adjunctive stent placement. The patency rates of 80–90% after 5 years that have been reported for short iliac stenoses are comparable to surgical results.

The question, whether or not all iliac stenoses should undergo stent treatment has been addressed in the Dutch Iliac Stent Trial. 279 patients with short iliac artery stenosis were randomly assigned to direct stent placement or primary angioplasty with subsequent stent placement in case of a residual mean pressure gradient >10 mmHg across the treated site (stent frequency in this group: 43%). As there were no substantial differences in technical results and clinical outcomes of the two treatment strategies both at short-term and long-term follow-up, provisional stenting in case of an insufficient angioplasty result can be considered the state of the art in the treatment of iliac artery stenoses.

To optimize and maintain international medical standards in the management of PAOD, a consensus expert opinion of key professional societies, the TransAtlantic Inter-Society Consensus (TASC) Working Group, has developed a consensus document. These recommendations of the TASC attempted to define a treatment of choice, depending on the morphologic

> **Contents DVD**
> 1. Stent-supported reconstruction of the aortic bifurcation (05:26 min)
> 2. Reconstruction of the aortic bifurcation with kissing stents (06:25 min)
> 3. Recanalization of a right common iliac artery occlusion (13:33 min)
> 4. Recanalization of a right external iliac artery occlusion (10:34 min)

stratification of iliac lesions *(Table 1)*. Thus, PTA is generally considered for more focal disease (type A and B lesion). For diffuse, extensive, complex multi-level, multifocal, or totally occluded atherosclerotic segments of the iliac arteries (type C and D lesion), TASC recommends surgery as the procedure of choice.

These recommendations may be a good guide for an institution with a low volume of interventions or during the initial phase starting the peripheral program. Completed in the middle of 1999, the consensus process represented, of course, the most up-to-date view at that time. However, in the last 4 years the development of new endovascular devices and stents has been proceeded extremely fast. For experienced and well-skilled interventionalists today the length and morphology of iliac lesions have less influence on technical success and long-time results. Therefore, the TASC recommendations are presently of limited value.

TABLE 1. *TASC recommendations for the treatment of iliac lesions.*
CFA: common femoral artery;
CIA: common iliac artery;
EIA: external iliac artery;
TASC: TransAtlantic Inter-Society Consensus.

TABLE 1.

Endovascular procedure is the treatment of choice for type A lesions, and surgery is the procedure of choice for type D lesions. More evidence is needed to make any firm recommendations about the best treatment for type B and C lesions.

TASC type A iliac lesions
- Single stenosis <3 cm of the CIA or EIA (unilateral/bilateral)

TASC type B iliac lesions
- Single stenosis 3 – 10 cm in length, not extending into the CFA
- Total of two stenoses <5 cm long in the CIA and/or EIA and not extending into the CFA
- Unilateral CIA occlusions

TASC type C iliac lesions
- Bilateral 5 – 10 cm long stenoses in the CIA and/or EIA and not extending into the CFA
- Unilateral EIA occlusion not extending into the CFA
- Unilateral EIA occlusion extending into the CFA
- Bilateral CIA occlusion

TASC type D iliac lesions
- Diffuse multiple unilateral stenoses involving the CIA, EIA, and CFA (usually >10 cm)
- Unilateral occlusion involving both the CIA and EIA
- Bilateral EIA occlusions
- Diffuse disease involving the aorta and both iliac arteries
- Iliac stenoses in a patient with an abdominal aortic aneurysm or other lesion requiring aortic or iliac surgery

Clinical Manifestation and Noninvasive Workup

Lifestyle-limiting claudication is the leading presenting symptom of patients with lower limb arterial obstructions. Exercise-induced pain in the calf is typically found in patients with femoral obstructions, whereas the complaints of patients with predominantly aortoiliac disease may be more unspecific with ischemic pain in the thigh during walking or even pain in the back and the hips. As these complaints may occur during exercise as well as at rest, they are frequently misdiagnosed as orthopedic or ischiadic problems.

After clinical examination, all patients should undergo standardized treadmill test for objective measurement of the walking capacity as well as calculation of the Ankle-Brachial Index (ABI) at rest and after exercise. Color-coded duplex sonography is less valuable for the detection of obstructions in the iliac arteries by direct imaging. In most cases, it is also impossible to estimate the collateralization of iliac obstructions. Otherwise, indirect Doppler criteria including the pattern of Doppler spectrum and the peak flow velocity in the common femoral artery may indicate an upstreamed iliac artery lesion (see Chapter 1, Figure 2). Furthermore, coexistent obstructions in the femoropopliteal or infrapopliteal arteries can be reliably diagnosed using duplex sonography.

Spiral computed tomography (CT) imaging and magnetic resonance angiography (MRA) may provide – particularly in case of total occlusions of the aortoiliac segment – valuable additional information about the presence of thrombus, the underlying atherosclerotic obstructions, and the degree of calcification.

Angiography

In all cases with unclear arterial obstructions, an intraarterial angiography will follow the noninvasive workup. In most of the cases, diagnostic angiography can be performed on an outpatient basis using 4-F diagnostic catheters. For imaging of the infrarenal aorta, the aortic bifurcation and the pelvic arteries, mechanical injection of contrast media should be performed (20–25 ml contrast media, flow ~ 15 ml/s).

Due to the anatomic location and the frequent turtuosity of the iliac arteries, a single posterior-anterior projection may be insufficient. Additional lateral views may be helpful for optimal imaging of specific arterial segments.

> **TIPS AND TRICKS**
>
> ■ *In case of unspecific complaints in the hip and/or thigh rule out a pelvic artery obstruction as the underlying cause.*
>
> ■ *Visualization of the external / internal iliac artery bifurcation: 30–45° contralateral angulation.*
>
> ■ *Visualization of the femoral bifurcation: 30–45° ipsilateral angulation.*

Devices' choice – Stent

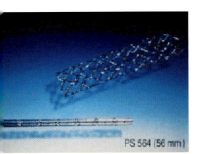

Figure 1. *Palmaz stent.*

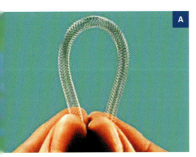

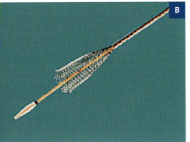

Figures 2a and 2b. *Wallstent (a) and application system (b).*

Endoluminal stents for peripheral applications can be broadly classified into two conceptionally different types: balloon-expandable and self-expanding devices.

Balloon-Expandable Stents

The Palmaz stent *(Figure 1)* is the prototype of balloon-expandable stents for implantation in the iliac arteries. This stent is, essentially, a laser-cut slotted tube of stainless steel. For implantation, the stent is hand-crimped on a suitably sized balloon catheter. Important characteristics of this balloon-expandable stent include its high radial force which makes it the preferred choice for eccentric, heavily calcified lesions. The intensive radiopacity allows a precise placement with minimal foreshortening which favors its application for ostial lesions. Furthermore, the stent allows further expansion after the initial deployment through the use of incrementally larger balloons.

Meanwhile, a variety of balloon-expandable stents have been developed. Modifications in stent design were made in order to improve the flexibility of the stent while maintaining the outstanding radial force of stainless-steel balloon-expandable stents. Furthermore, all stents are now available in a pre-mounted form on a PTA catheter, which improves the handling of the device during implantation. Generally, all of these endoprostheses are well applicable to iliac arteries, without any of the stent designs showing a clear advantage. Although crossover implantation is possible in the majority of the cases, the flexibility of all balloon-expandable stents remains limited.

Self-Expanding Stents

The most distinguishing feature between self-expanding and balloon-expandable devices is the higher flexibility of all self-expanding stent designs, which facilitates crossover implantation as well as the application in very tortuous iliac vessels. The prototype is the Wallstent *(Figure 2a)*, which is based on a wire mesh made from spring-like stainless-steel monofilaments. For implantation, the stent is contained in an application system *(Figure 2b)*. When released, the stent recoils to its preset diameter. During that process, a significant foreshortening of the endoprosthesis up to one third of the unconstrained state occurs. Since the deployment sometimes may become imprecise, this stent design is not recommendable for ostial lesions or stenting close to side branches. Furthermore, the radial force of self-expanding stents is considerably lower than that of balloon-expandable endoprostheses which may limit their use in highly calcified lesions.

While the self-expanding characteristics of the Wallstent are based on its spring-like stainless steel monofilaments, another concept of self-expanding is that the stent employs the thermal memory characteristics of nitinol. Nitinol is an elastic intermetallic alloy of nickel and titanium with a so-called thermal shape memory. Preshaped at high temperatures to its nominal dimension, the stent is soft and deformable when cooled. When exposed to body temperature during deployment, the stent self-expands rapidly to its nominal diameter. Currently, several nitinol stents are available. The radial stiffness of some of these stents seems to be superior to the Wallstent while maintaining a high flexibility. Furthermore, less foreshortening occurs which makes the implantation more predictable. Compared to the Wallstent,

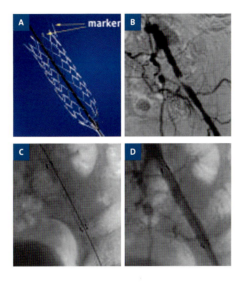

nitinol stents are generally much less visible. To enhance visibility, several stents have highly radiopaque markers at the edge of the stent *(Figure 3a)*. After releasing the stent, postdilatation is mostly necessary to achieve a full adaptation of the stent to the vessel wall and, of course, a good angiographic result *(Figures 3b to 3d)*. Expanding the nitinol stents further then their nominal diameter will lead to stent deformation and has to be avoided.

FIGURES 3A TO 3D.

a) Self-expanding nitinol stent with radiopaque edges (Luminexx, Bard Access Systems, Salt Lake City, UT, USA).
b) High-grade stenosis of the left external iliac artery.
c) After direct stenting, remaining relevant narrowing of the vessel. Very good visibility due to the highly radiopaque stent edges.
d) Final result after post-dilatation (balloon diameter 7 mm).

Procedure Techniques

Retrograde Iliac Approach

In most of the cases, iliac artery interventions can be performed using the ipsilateral retrograde access. After local anesthesia of the puncture site, a long (25 cm) hemostatic introducer sheath (in most of the cases 6–7 F) is placed. Routinely, 5,000 IU of heparin are administered before the intervention.

The initial passage of the iliac artery stenosis *(Figure 4a)* can be performed using a standard 0.018" guide wire, however, also a soft angle-tipped 0.035" hydrophilic guide wire (Terumo, Tokyo, Japan) has been proven effective in most of the cases.

For PTA of the stenosis, the dimensions of the balloon should be chosen according to the length of the lesion

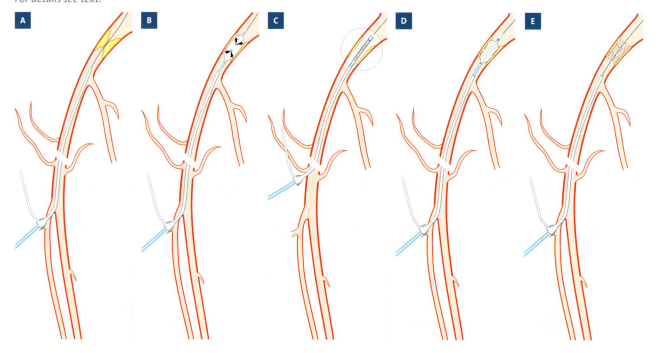

FIGURES 4A TO 4E.
Retrograde iliac stent placement.
For details see text.

(standard balloon length 20–40 mm) and by comparison with the proximal and distal reference segment (mostly 7–10 mm for the common iliac artery, 6–8 mm for the external iliac artery). If a primary stent implantation is considered, predilatation of the stenosis should be performed with an undersized balloon and low dilatation pressure *(Figure 4b)*.

Usually, a balloon-expandable stent will be a good choice for retrograde implantation, as it allows precise placement and has the potential to further expand with larger balloons, if necessary. A self-expanding stent may be considered for long, uncalcified, non-ostial lesions. For implantation of the balloon-expandable stent, a long introducer sheath should be advanced through the lesion before delivery of the stent to avoid potential friction between stent and obstruction followed by dislodgment of the stent. After stent positioning *(Figure 4c)*, the sheath will be withdrawn to allow stent deployment *(Figure 4d)*. Depending on the resistance of the stenosis, the implantation pressure usually ranges between 8–12 atm with an inflation time of 30–60 s. To avoid vessel rupture, the diameter of the balloon for stent placement should be chosen according to the diameter of the proximal or distal reference vessel segment. The result of the intervention *(Figure 4e)* should be controlled angiographically using two different projections. Furthermore, the residual translesion pressure gradient can be measured using the long introducer sheath. In case of insufficient stent expansion, additional dilatations with larger balloons may be performed. However, overdilatation should always be avoided given the risk of a vessel rupture.

> **TIPS AND TRICKS**
>
> ▪ *Sizing of balloon-expandable stents should be made according to the reference vessel diameter. Diameter of self-expanding stents should be chosen 1–2 mm larger than the reference vessel diameter.*
>
> ▪ *If the patient complains of pain during inflation of the balloon in the iliac artery, stop immediately; a perforation or rupture may be imminent.*

Crossover approach

Crossover placement of self-expanding stents is usually easy, whereas crossover implantation of more rigid balloon-expandable stents is technically more challenging and requires the use of crossover sheaths (Cook, Bjaeverskov, Denmark, or a 7-F Super Arrow-Flex Sheath, Arrow, Reading, USA). Due to a higher kinkability, a Brite Tip sheath (Cordis, Miami, USA) is only suitable in the case of a nonangulated bifurcation. Alternatively, a suitably sized guiding catheter can be used as crossover system.

Step-by-step crossover procedure: first, a soft hydrophilic guide wire is navigated in crossover position with the help of a suitably shaped 5-F diagnostic catheter (JR5, Cobra, Hook, Shepherd's Hook) *(Figure 5a-c)*. Second, the catheter is gently advanced over the guide wire, which is then exchanged against a stiff wire (Amplatz, ultrastiff, Boston Sc., or a Hi-Torque Supracore 0.035" guide wire, Guidant, Santa Clara, USA). The stiff wire opens the angle of the aortic bifurcation and facilitates placement of the crossover sheath. After optional predilatation *(Figure 5d)* the balloon catheter with the mounted stent is advanced within the sheath up to the aortic bifurcation.

To bring the stent around the bifurcation, it may be necessary to push the crossover sheath forward until the end of the endoprosthesis, which is passively moving within the sheath, reaches the contralateral common iliac artery *(Figure 5e)*. From this position, the

FIGURES 5A TO 5F.
Crossover stent placement. For details see text.

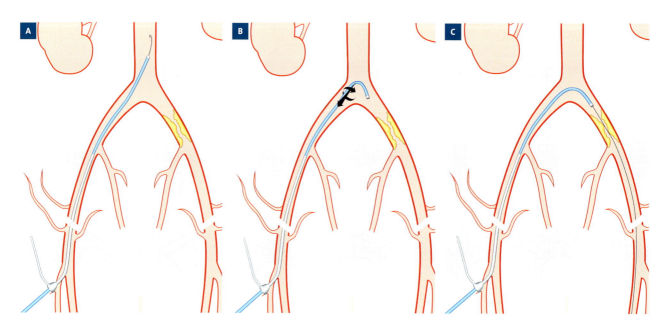

balloon catheter can be further advanced without moving the sheath. After correct positioning, the stent is implanted as described above *(Figure 5f)*.

Transbrachial approach

The brachial artery access is an important alternative vascular access and may be used particularly in the case of severe bilateral iliac obstructions. To avoid crossing of the aortic arch with the attendant risk of cerebral embolization and to have a more direct access to the descending aorta, the left brachial approach should be preferred, whenever possible. By advancing a 90 cm long shuttle introducer (Flexor Check-Flo Performer, Cook, Bjaeverskov, Denmark) in front of the bifurcation of the abdominal aorta, the iliac arteries are directly accessible. With this very stable access, every kind of manipulation to the iliac arteries is possible, and even bilateral lesions can be treated in one session.

The balloon catheter with the pre-mounted stent is advanced within the sheath down to the aortic bifurcation. For implantation of the stent, the long introducer sheath will be advanced into the origin of the appropriate common iliac artery. Then, the balloon catheter can be further pushed without moving the sheath. After correct positioning, the stent is implanted as described above.

> **TIPS AND TRICKS**
>
> ▪ *Remove the brachial sheath immediately after the procedure to avoid thrombotic complications of the puncture site.*

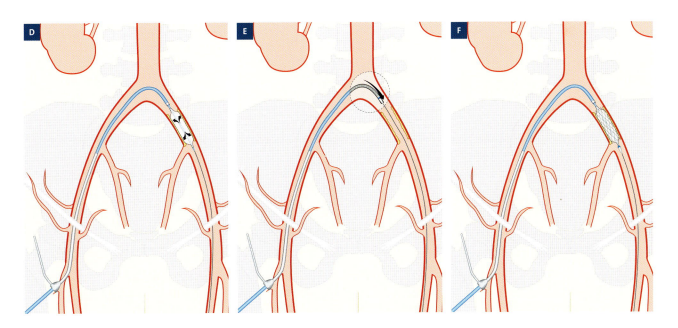

Specific cases

Chronic Iliac Artery Occlusions

Access Method and Lesion Crossing

The percutaneous treatment of iliac artery stenoses is mostly a relatively simple procedure, whereas the recanalization of a totally occluded iliac artery is technically demanding. Possible approaches to the occlusion include the retrograde, the crossover and the brachial access. Although frequently used, the ipsilateral retrograde approach has the disadvantage of a more difficult arterial puncture distal to the occluded segment. Furthermore, it may be difficult to navigate the guide wire intraluminally through the occlusion, which may result in extensive dissection of the vessel wall, which – particularly in the region of the aortic bifurcation – may cause significant problems. In our practice, the crossover is the preferred primary access for recanalization of total occlusions.

After retrograde puncture and sheath placement into the contralateral common femoral artery, a 5-F guiding catheter (Hook or Shepherd's Hook) is positioned at the aortic bifurcation. The occlusion is initially passed with a stiff 0.035" hydrophilic guide wire (angled tip, Terumo, Tokyo, Japan), which is finally placed into the common femoral artery *(Figure 6a)*.

> **TIPS AND TRICKS**
>
> - Always consider an antegrade approach to the lesion via crossover or brachial approach with a long sheath as the initial option for total iliac artery occlusions.

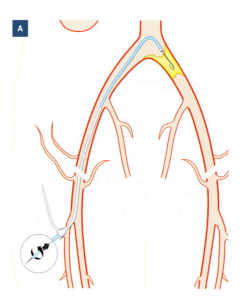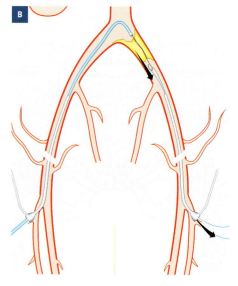

FIGURES 6A AND 6B.
Recanalization of the iliac occlusions, crossover. For details see text.

Using the guide wire as a marker, the ipsilateral common femoral artery is punctured under fluoroscopic control, and a second 8-F introducer sheath is placed. Using an angled wire loop, introduced through the ipsilateral sheath, the tip of the guide wire in crossover position is snared and retrieved out of the sheath *(Figure 6b)*. The following steps of the procedure are performed using this retrograde access as described in Figure 4.

Endoprosthesis Implantation

After predilatation of the occluded region with an undersized balloon, primary stent implantation is performed in all cases. The choice of the stent device is based on the same considerations as described for iliac artery stenoses. Balloon-expandable stents will be preferred for the ostium of the common or external iliac artery, whereas self expanding-stents can be used to stabilize longer, less calcified vessel segments *(Figure 7)*.

Reconstruction of the Aortoiliac Bifurcation

Although the clinical introduction of endovascular stents has contributed to an expansion of indications for minimally invasive endovascular procedures, there is only limited experience with PTA for the treatment of bilateral iliac obstructions involving the aortic bifurcations. The potential of contralateral embolism or contralateral iliac artery occlusion due to dislodgment of atherosclerotic or thrombotic material during unilateral PTA has prevented the common use of interventional techniques in this vessel segment. To avoid such complications, the kissing balloon technique was developed for bilateral simultaneous angioplasty and stent implantation into the common iliac arteries and the distal abdominal aorta *(Figure 8)*.

Access Method and Lesion Crossing

The standard approach for bilateral iliac artery stenoses is the retrograde technique. After bilateral sheath placement (6–8 F), on each side, an 0.018" guide wire is navigated through the lesion.

> **TIPS AND TRICKS**
>
> ■ *For reconstruction of the aortic bifurcation the use of balloon-expandable stents with a high radial force is recommended.*
>
> ■ *For lesions with severe differences in proximal and distal reference vessel diameter and lesions close to the inguinal ligament use self-expanding stents.*

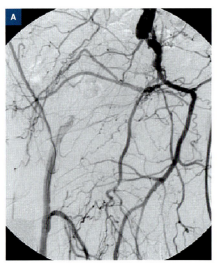 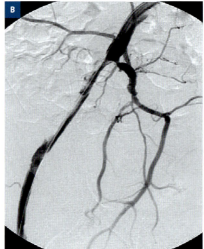 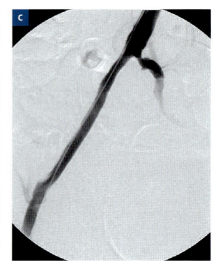

Figures 7a to 7c.
a) Chronic total occlusion of the right external iliac artery.
b) Primary channel after recanalization with a stiff hydrophilic guide wire and predilatation with a 5-mm balloon.
c) Final result after implantation of a self-expanding stent (Dynalink™ 8.0/100 mm) and postdilatation of the stent with a 6-mm balloon (Sailor™ 6.0/80 mm).

Dilatation Process, Endoprosthesis Implantation

Simultaneous predilatations with undersized balloons are performed using the kissing balloon technique. For this indication, only balloon-expandable stents with a high radial force can be recommended, as ostial lesions of the common iliac arteries are mostly very calcified. Furthermore, a precise placement of the stents at the aortic bifurcation is essential for reconstruction of the aortoiliac segment. For optimal reconstruction of the aortoiliac segment, the stents should extend slightly (about 2 mm) into the lumen of the aorta to prevent plaque protrusion at the bifurcation. In case of more extensive disease in the aorta itself, separate deployment of a balloon-expandable stent (Palmaz stent) in the aorta may have to precede the deployment of kissing iliac stents.

Large aortic balloons with diameters between 20 and 25 mm allow only low-pressure inflations (2–4 atm), and thus are only applicable to the initial stent deployment. If necessary, simultaneous dilatation of the aortic stent with two balloons (diameter 8–10 mm) should be performed to achieve an optimal expansion of the stent.

Postprocedural Treatment

During intervention, all patients receive 5,000–10,000 IU heparin intraarterially. A combination of acetylsalicylic acid (ASA) (100 mg/d) and clopidogrel 75 mg/d or ticlopidine (250 mg b.i.d. for 4 weeks) is given to all patients.

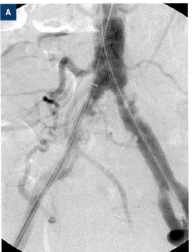 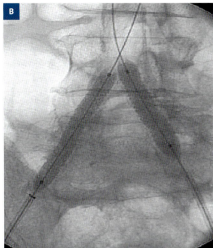 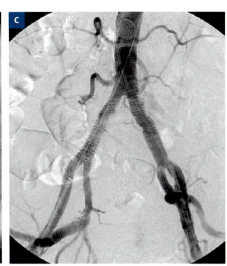

FIGURES 8A TO 8C.
a) Bilateral high-grade ostial stenosis of the common iliac arteries (CIA).
b) Simultaneous direct stenting of the stenotic lesions in "kissing balloon technique", using balloon-expandable stents (Omnilink™ 8.0/56 mm for right CIA and Omnilink™ 10.0/38 mm for left CIA).
c) Final result after postdilatation of the stents likewise in "kissing balloon technique" (Sailor Plus™ 9.0/40 mm for right CIA and Sailor Plus™ 10.0/40 mm for left CIA).

Summary of Outcome Results

Iliac Artery Stenoses

PTA of atherosclerotic iliac artery stenosis is an effective and established method of recanalization with low complication rates and long-term results approaching surgical bypass procedure outcomes. Since the success of iliac angioplasty is related to factors such as length, eccentricity, calcification of the lesion, and the presence of occlusions or stenoses, obstructions of the pelvic arteries are classified into four categories. Generally, the best results, with technical success rates of > 95% and 5-year patency rates of 80–90%, have been reported for short-segment stenosis.

Iliac Artery Occlusions

Compared to procedures treating nonocclusive stenoses, total occlusion recanalizations show a 10–15% lower success rate.

We analyzed the data of 212 patients with unilateral chronic iliac artery occlusions who were interventionally treated in our institution by angioplasty and primary stent implantation. A technical success could be achieved in 190 of the 212 patients (89.6%), associated with a marked clinical improvement by three or two grades according to the American Heart Association (AHA) guidelines in 112 (52.8%) and 67 cases (31.6%), respectively. The major complication rate in this series was 1.4%. Primary patency rates of 81.2% at 2 and 75.7% at 4 years demonstrate that this technique is a safe and effective treatment for patients with chronic iliac artery occlusions *(Table 2)*.

TABLE 2. *Treatment of total iliac artery occlusions. Comparison of interventional and surgical data from the literature. NA: not available; PTA: percutaneous transluminal angioplasty.*

TABLE 2.

Author	Patients (n)	Technical success (%)	Major complications[a] (%)	Minor complications[b] (%)	Primary patency (%)	Follow-up time (months)
Iliac stent studies						
Scheinert et al.	212	89.6	1.4	6.6	77.9	36
Vorwerk et al.	103	79.5	10.6	2	81[c]	36
Reyes et al.	59	92	8.5	5.1	73	24
Kim et al.	34	100	0	2.9	94	12
Iliac PTA studies						
Johnston et al.	82	81.7	8.4	6	66	36
Colapinto et al.	64	78	3.1	0	78	6–48
Gupta et al.	50	78.6	8.9	14.3	76	36

		Operative mortality (%)	Systemic morbidity (%)	Local morbidity (%)		
Aortoiliac bypass studies						
Szilagyi et al.	1,748	5	18.9	6	85.3	60
Nevelsteen et al.	912	5.5	8.6	9	88.9	60
Van den Akker et al.	518	3.3	NA	NA	86.5	60

[a] such as acute ischemia, distal embolism, dissections, vessel rupture and mortality
[b] puncture site complications including hematomas, false aneurysms, arteriovenous fistulas
[c] technical failures excluded

Obstructions of the Aortoiliac Bifurcation and Infrarenal Aorta

Until recently, the experience with PTA for complex bilateral aortoiliac obstructions is limited and has been reported only sporadically and for small numbers of patients. In 1999, we published a series of 48 patients with obstructions of the aortoiliac segments which underwent kissing stent implantation. Stents were placed successfully and without complications in all patients. A clinical improvement by two to three grades according to the AHA criteria was observed in 41 and seven patients, respectively. The primary angiographic patency rate at 2 years was 86.8%. In three cases, significant restenoses were detected, which could be successfully treated by PTA *(Table 3)*.

TABLE 3.

Author	Patients (n)	Technical success (%)	Major complications (%)	Primary patency (%)	Follow-up (months)
Scheinert	48	100	0	87	24
Haulon	106	100	0	81 / 79	24 / 36
Mouanoutoua	50	100	4	92	20[a]

[a] mean follow-up

TABLE 3. *Stent-supported reconstruction of the aortoiliac bifurcation. Cumulative patency rates.*

References

1. Biamino G, Dörschel K, Harnoss BM, Kar H, Müller G. Experience in excimer laser photoablation of atherosclerotic plaques. In: Biamino G, Müller GJ, eds. Advances in laser medicine. First German Symposium on Laser Angioplasty. Berlin: Ecomed 1988:147–56.

2. Blum U, Gabelmann A, Redecker M, Noldge G, Dornberg W, Grosser G, Heiss W, Langer M. Percutaneous recanalization of iliac artery occlusions: results of a prospective study. Radiology 1993;189: 536–40.

3. Brothers TE, Greefield LJ. Long-term results of aorto-iliac reconstruction. J Vasc Interv Radiol 1990;1:49–55.

4. Colapinto RF, Stronell RD, Johnston WK. Transluminal angioplasty of complete iliac obstructions. AJR Am J Roentgenol 1986;146:859–62.

5. Cumberland DC, Sanborn TA, Tayler DI, Moore DJ, Welsh CL, Greenfield AJ, Guben JK, Ryan TJ. Percutaneous laser thermal angioplasty: initial clinical results with a laser probe in total peripheral artery occlusions. Lancet 1986;1457–9.

6. Gupta AK, Ravimandalam K, Rao VR, Joseph S, Unni M, Rao AS, Neelkandhan KS. Total occlusion of iliac arteries: results of balloon angioplasty. Cardiovasc Intervent Radiol 1993;16:165–77.

7. Haulon S, Mounier-Vehier C, Gaxotte V, Koussa M, Lions C, Haouari BA, Beregi JP. Percutaneous reconstruction of the aortoiliac bifurcation with the "kissing stents" technique: long-term follow-up in 106 patients: J Endovasc Ther 2002;9:363–8.

8. Hausegger KA, Lammer J, Klein G, Fluckiger E, Pilger E, Lafer M. Perkutane Rekanalisation von Beckenarterienverschlüssen: Fibrinolyse, PTA, Stents. Fortschr Roentgenstr 1991;155:550–5.

9. Henry M, Amor M, Ethevenot G, Henry I, Amicabile C, Beron R, Mentre B, Allaoui M, Touchot N. Palmaz stent placement in iliac and femoropopliteal arteries: primary and secondary patency in 310 patients with 2–4 year follow-up. Radiology 1995;197:167–74.

10. Johnston KW. Iliac arteries: reanalysis of results of balloon angioplasty. Radiology 1993;186:207–12.

11. Kannel WB, Skinner JJ Jr, Schwartz MJ, Shurtleff D. Intermittent claudication: incidence in the Framingham Study. Circulation 1970;41:875–83.

12. Kim JK, Kim YH, Chung SY, Kang HK. Primary stent placement for recanalization of iliac artery occlusions using a self-expanding spiral stent. Cardiovasc Intervent Radiol 1999;22:278–81.

13. Küffer G, Spengler F, Steckmeier B. Percutaneous reconstruction of the aortic bifurcation with Palmaz stents: case report. Cardiovasc Intervent Radiol 1991;14: 170–2.

14. Management of peripheral arterial disease (PAD). TransAtlantic Inter-Society Consensus (TASC). J Vasc Surg 2000;31:Suppl: 1–296.

15. Morag G, Rubinstein Z, Kessler A, Schneiderman J, Levinkopf M, Bass A. Percutaneous transluminal angioplasty of the distal abdominal aorta and its bifurcation. Cardiovasc Intervent Radiol 1987;10:129–33.

16. Murphy KD, Encarnacion CE, Le VA, Palmaz JC. Iliac artery stent placement with the Palmaz stent: follow-up study. J Vasc Interv Radiol 1995;6:321–9.

17. Mouanoutoua M, Maddikunta R, Allaqaband S, Gupta A, Shalev Y, Tumuluri R, Bajwa T. Endovascular intervention of aortoiliac occlusive disease in high-risk patients using the kissing stents technique: long-term results. Cathet Cardiovasc Interv 2003;60:320–6.

18. Nevelsteen A, Wouters L, Suy R. Long-term patency of the aortofemoral Dacron graft: a graft limb related study over a 25-years period. J Cardiovasc Surg (Torino) 1991;32:174–80.

19. Pentecost MJ, Criqui MH, Dorros G, Goldstone J, Johnston W, Martin EC, Ring EJ, Spies JB. Guidelines for peripheral percutaneous transluminal angioplasty of the abdominal aorta and lower extremity vessels. Circulation 1994;89:511–31.

20. Reyes R, Maynar M, Lopera J, Ferral H, Gorriz E, Carreira J, Castaneda WR. Treatment of chronic iliac artery occlusions with guide wire recanalization and primary stent placement. J Vasc Interv Radiol 1997;8: 1049–55.

21. Scheinert D, Schröder M, Balzer JO, Steinkamp H, Biamino G. Stent-supported reconstruction of the aorto-iliac bifurcation with the kissing balloon technique. Circulation 1999;100 Suppl II 295–300.

22. Scheinert D, Schroeder M, Ludwig J, Bräunlich S, Möckel M, Flachskampf FA, Balzer JO, Biamino G. Stent-supported recanalization of chronic iliac artery occlusions. Am J Med 2001;110:708–15.

23. Standards of Practice Committee of the Society of Cardiovascular and Interventional Radiology. Guidelines for percutaneous transluminal angioplasty. Radiology 1990;177:619–26.

24. Sullivan TM, Childs MB, Bacharach JM, Gray BH, Piedmonte MR. Percutaneous transluminal angioplasty and primary stenting of the iliac arteries in 288 patients. J Vasc Surg 1997;25:829–38.

25. Szilagyi DE, Elliott JP Jr, SmithRF, Reddy DJ, McPharlin M. A thirty-year survey of the reconstructive surgical treatment of aortoiliac occlusive disease. J Vasc Surg 1986;3:421–36.

26. Tegtmeyer CJ, Hartwell GD, Selby JB, Robertson R, Kron IL, Tribble CG. Results and complications of angioplasty in aorto-iliac disease. Circulation 1991;83:Suppl I:I-53–60.

27. Tegtmeyer CJ, Wellons HA, Thompson RN. Balloon dilatation of the abdominal aorta. JAMA 1980;244:2626–37.

28. Tetteroo E, van der Graaf Y, Bosch JL, van Engelen AD, Hunink MG, Eikelboom BC, Mali WP. Randomised comparison of primary stent placement versus primary angioplasty followed by selective stent placement in patients with iliac artery occlusive disease. Dutch Iliac Stent Trial Study Group. Lancet 1998;351:1153–9.

29. Van den Akker PJ, Van Schilfgaarde R, Brand R, Hajo von Bockel J, Terpstra JL. Long-term results of prosthetic reconstruction for obstructive aortoiliac disease. Eur J Vasc Surg 1992;6:53–61.

30. Velasquez G, Castanbeda-Zuniga W, Formanek A. Non-surgical aortoplasty in Leriche syndrome. Radiology 1980;134:359–60.

31. Vorwerk D, Günther RW, Schürmann K, Wendt G. Aortic and iliac stenoses: follow-up results of stent placement after insufficient balloon angioplasty in 118 cases. Radiology 1996;198:45–8.

32. Vorwerk D, Günther RW, Schürmann K, Wendt G, Peters I. Primary stent placement for chronic iliac artery occlusions: follow-up results in 103 patients. Radiology 1995;194:745–9.

33. Vries SO de, Hunink MGM. Results of aortic bifurcation grafts for aorto-iliac occlusive disease: a meta-analysis. J Vasc Surg 1997;26:558–69.

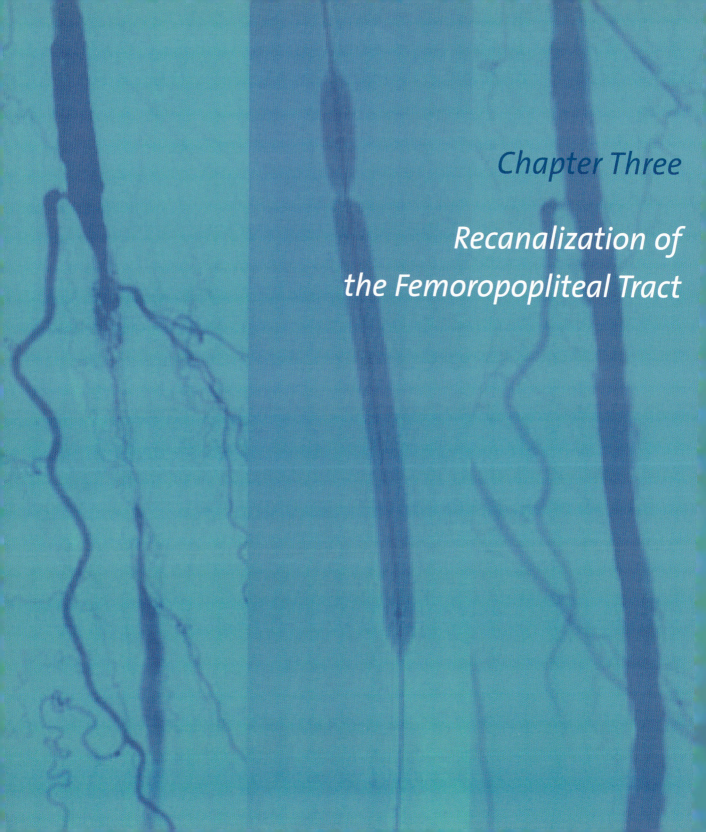

Chapter Three

Recanalization of the Femoropopliteal Tract

Introduction

Analyzing the distribution of peripheral arterial obstructive disease (PAOD), >50% of all lesions are localized in the femoropopliteal tract. Occlusions predominate by a factor of at least 3 over stenoses in this arterial segment. Furthermore, most femoropopliteal occlusions are extensive and there is often coexistent multilevel atherosclerotic disease.

In this segment percutaneous transluminal angioplasty (PTA) is normally recommended as the treatment of choice for short stenoses and occlusions. By contrast, long chronic occlusions of the superficial femoral artery (SFA) are still mainly considered for vascular surgery. However, bypass grafting is associated with a considerable procedure-related morbidity and mortality.

Therefore, surgical intervention is usually reserved for patients with ischemic rest pain or very advanced claudication. Consequently, many patients with long chronic SFA disease, although in a state of relevant discomfort, remain untreated. A walking program is often recommended. However, even in supervised exercise programs only 20–25% of PAOD patients can be included and the benefit tends to be short-lived after completion of the supervision.

Percutaneous revascularization techniques permit a lower threshold for interventions than has been traditionally practiced for surgical procedures, but long-term results after recanalization of especially extensive obstructions of the SFA are sometimes unsatisfactory. Therefore, improvement and development of new techniques for endovascular recanalization are particularly desirable and discussed in this chapter.

Contents DVD

5. PTA of SFA stenoses (13:01 min)
10. Multilevel recanalization of left SFA and ATA (10:01 min)
6. Laser recanalization of a right SFA occlusion (05:59 min)
7. Endovascular atherectomy for SFA in-stent restenosis (06:21 min)
8. Subintimal recanalization with the Pioneer catheter (11:30 min)

Patient Selection and Diagnostic Methods

Chronic atherosclerotic obstructions of the SFA are the leading cause of lifestyle-limiting intermittent claudication. Patients typically complain of exercise-induced pain in the calf, which resolves after a few minutes of rest. Ischemic rest pain or nonhealing ulceration occurs only in a relatively small percentage of patients, mainly with multilevel disease.

Diagnostic Possibilities

Especially in the femoropopliteal tract, duplex sonography is highly effective for location of the lesion and differentiation between stenosis and total occlusion, and precise enough for planning the intervention. Diagnostic angiography with depiction of the abdominal aorta, pelvic and leg arteries can be part of the endovascular procedure. Preinterventional magnetic resonance angiography is practical in patients with renal insufficiency. On this basis, angiography can be limited to the site of the lesion and the intervention can be performed with a minimal amount of contrast media (normally < 50 ml).

TIPS AND TRICKS

- *Duplex sonography is sufficient for the preinterventional workup of patients with SFA lesions.*

Access to Femoropopliteal Lesions

In our opinion, the crossover approach from the contralateral common femoral artery (CFA) can be considered the standard technique for femoropopliteal interventions. As compared to the antegrade access, the retrograde puncture is much easier achieved and subsequent complications including hemorrhage from the access site are rare. Furthermore, with this technique postinterventional flow reduction during manual compression and subsequent bandage is applied to the contralateral leg; thus, the flow in the recanalized vessel segment is not reduced, which subsequently may contribute to the reduction of early thrombotic reocclusions. Another main advantage in contrast to the antegrade access is that also very proximal lesions of the SFA can be treated.

After insertion of a short 5-F sheath, the crossover navigation of the guide wire is easily achieved using a right Judgkins catheter, an IMA (internal mammary artery) or Cobra catheter *(Figure 1a)* or in severely angulated bifurcations a Hook *(Figure 1b)*, a Shepherd's Hook *(Figure 1c)* or an Omni Selective

Recanalization of the Femoropopliteal Tract

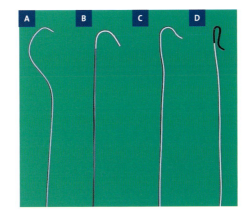

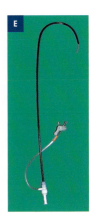

catheter *(Figure 1d)* or even a pigtail catheter. The guide wire of choice is the 0.035" soft-angled Terumo wire (Terumo, Tokyo, Japan). After the guide wire and the diagnostic catheter are positioned in the contralateral CFA, a stiffer 0.035" guide wire (e.g., the Supracore 190 cm; Guidant, Saint Paul, MN, USA) is exchanged for the Terumo wire and a crossover sheath (Cook *[Figure 1e]* or Arrow) is inserted *(Figure 2)*. Usually, a 6-F sheath can be chosen, since balloons and most of the available self-expanding nitinol stents are now 6-F-compatible. However, especially in highly calcified or severely angulated bifurcations it is advisable to use a larger sheath (7 F or even 8 F) to avoid kinking and reduce friction of the interventional instruments within the sheath.

In cases, where a crossover recanalization has failed or cannot be performed due to specific anatomic situations (e.g., stents in the region of the aortic bifurcation or aortoiliac prosthesis), the antegrade femoral approach is an alternative technique except for very proximal lesions of the SFA. It should also be preferred in very caicified

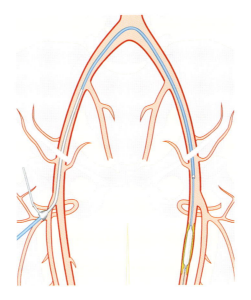

and significantly kinked pelvic arteries, which make precise navigation of the guide wires, especially in calcified occlusions of the SFA, difficult or impossible.

Although a high puncture of the CFA is recommended to have enough space for navigation of the guide wire into the SFA, suprainguinal puncture should be avoided due to the risk of

FIGURES 1A TO 1E.
Different catheters for achieving a crossover approach.
a) Cobra catheter.
b) Hook catheter.
c) Shepherd's Hook catheter.
d) Omni Selective catheter.
e) A 7-F crossover sheath (Cook).

FIGURE 2.
Crossover technique for recanalization of the femoropopliteal tract.

TIPS AND TRICKS

■ *First-choice access for recanalization of the SFA is the crossover approach.*

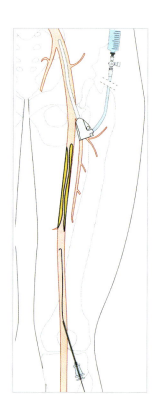

FIGURE 4. *Popliteal puncture.*

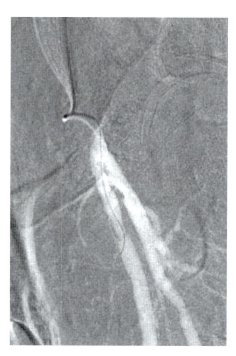

FIGURE 3. *A lateral angulation and a road map are helpful during antegrade puncture.*

retroperitoneal hemorrhage. Therefore, a rather steep puncture has to be performed in many cases. If the guide wire is introduced into the deep femoral artery, a 4-F dilator can be inserted and is pulled back into the CFA during continuous contrast injection, where an angulated Terumo wire is used for navigation into the SFA. A lateral projection of the femoral bifurcation is helpful in this situation *(Figure 3)*.

Recanalization of femoropopliteal occlusions using the transpopliteal technique can be considered a salvage technique after failed crossover attempts. Only patients with a patent proximal popliteal and distal femoral artery as well as a sufficient peripheral runoff can be considered for this approach. To achieve a safe puncture of the popliteal artery, first a 4-F sheath is placed retrograde into the ipsilateral CFA. The patient is then turned to a prone position. The popliteal puncture is performed with the assistance of road-map fluoroscopy by injection of contrast media through the 4-F sheath *(Figure 4)*. The needle often has to be introduced in a steep angle (70–80°) and up to 5 cm in depth. The wire for sheath insertion (normally a 6-F/12-cm sheath) should not be removed before a guide wire for recanalization is introduced into the artery, otherwise the sheath might kink due to the steep puncture, making further wire introduction difficult. This approach is successful in up to 80% after formerly failed antegrade recanalization attempts of SFA occlusions.

If none of the above access sites seems suitable, a brachial approach can be chosen. A 90 cm long 6- or 7-F sheath is recommended for sufficient support during the intervention. For distal lesions balloons (Sailor and Submarine, Invatec) and stents (Optimed) with a working length of 150 cm are available.

Lesion Crossing

The initial passage of femoropopliteal stenoses can be performed using a standard 0.018" guide wire. Our first choice is the V18-control-wire (Boston Scientific), which, due to a stiff body and a hydrophilic tip, provides a good steerability and low friction for an intraluminal passage of stenoses and even total occlusions. In case of failed passage of occlusions an angled-tipped 0.035" stiff hydrophilic guide wire (Terumo) is recommended. A diagnostic multipurpose catheter (4 F or 5 F) improves the steerability of the guide wire and provides additional support for lesion crossing. Alternatively, a laser catheter (Spectranetics) can be used for crossing and additional debulking of stenoses or total occlusions of the SFA (see below).

> **TIPS AND TRICKS**
>
> ■ Hydrophilic coated 0.018" and 0.035" guide wires or laser catheters are recommended for passage of total occlusions of the SFA.

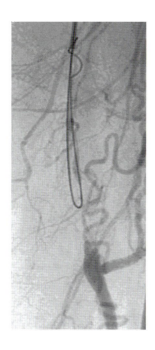

FIGURE 5. *Loop of the Terumo wire during recanalization of a total occlusion indicating a subintimal track.*

In older chronic occlusions initial passage of the wire into the lesion can be a difficult task. Forceful pressing of a guiding catheter into the occlusion for better support and repeat attempts with an angled or straight Terumo wire or even a cautious strike with the very stiff false end of the Terumo wire, alternatively a first laser cut without wire guidance will lead to a wire entrance into the occlusion in nearly all cases. For further passage of the occlusion, the Terumo wire is allowed to form a loop, indicating a subintimal track of the guide wire (Figure 5). This will occur in a high percentage of cases in chronic long occlusions. Alternatively, using the so-called percutaneous intended extraluminal (subintimal) recanalization

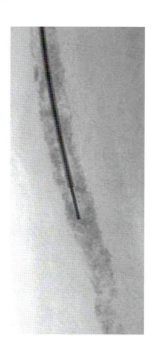

FIGURE 6. *Very stiff end of the Terumo wire during recanalization of a highly calcified occlusion.*

(PIER), the wire is directed subintimal at the very beginning of the occlusion by using an angulated support catheter. In heavily calcified occlusions wire passage can be very difficult. In this situation a cautious continuation of the recanalization with the false end of a Terumo wire for a short distance can be successful *(Figure 6)*.

To achieve reentry into the true lumen of the patent arterial segment distal to the occlusion, cautious probing with the wire tip is recommended to avoid further dissection of the artery into the healthy segment. The use of different guiding catheters and guide wires with straight and angled tips can be successful in this situation (e.g., 4-F or 5-F Glide catheter, angled or straight tip [Terumo], 5-F vertebral catheter; *Figure 7*).

However, inability to reenter the true lumen must be expected in up to 20% of total occlusions. According to our experience, the only predictor of failure is the degree of calcification. A transpopliteal approach can be an option in this situation. A new device, the Pioneer catheter (Medtronic, Santa Rosa, CA, USA), offers a novel, very effective salvage technique to redirect the guide wire into the patent vessel distal to the SFA occlusion. It consists of a 6.2-F double-lumen monorail catheter, which tracks over a 0.014" guide wire. The second lumen of the catheter contains a curved puncture needle for penetration of the intimal membrane *(Figure 8)*, which allows advancement of a second 0.014" guide wire into the true vessel lumen *(Figure 9)*. Furthermore, the tip of the catheter contains an intravascular ultrasound (IVUS) transducer, which

Tips and Tricks

- *In case of difficulty to reenter the true lumen distal to an occlusion, avoid further dissection into the healthy arterial segment.*

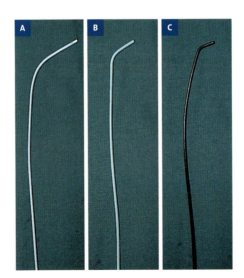

Figures 7a to 7c.
Different guiding catheters for reentry into the true lumen during recanalization of total occlusions.
a) Multipurpose catheter.
b) Vertebral catheter.
c) Angled Glide catheter.

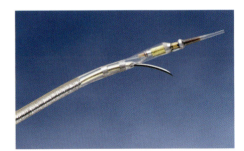

Figure 8. *Tip of the Pioneer catheter.*

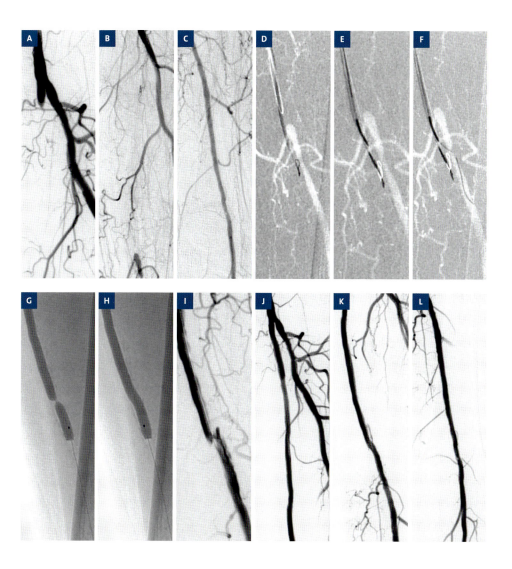

FIGURES 9A TO 9L.

a–c) Long occlusion of the left superficial femoral artery.
d) Failure to reenter the true lumen.
e) Pioneer catheter in place.
f) Puncture and wire passage into the true lumen.
g–i) Balloon dilatation and result.
j–l) Final result after stenting.

helps to direct the curved puncture needle into the true lumen. Using this device, recanalization success of long SFA occlusions reaches 100%. Furthermore, dissection distal to the reconstitution segment can be avoided, which can be of benefit if future bypass surgery becomes necessary.

Percutaneous Transluminal Balloon Angioplasty

TIPS AND TRICKS

- Low-profile balloons are recommended in very tight stenoses or occlusions.

The percutaneous transluminal balloon angioplasty can be considered the basic technique for femoropopliteal recanalization and can be recommended as a stand-alone procedure for treatment of short, focal femoropopliteal lesions in most of the cases.

The dimension of the balloon should be chosen according to the lesion length (standard balloon length 20–80 mm) and by comparison with the proximal and distal vessel segment (normally 5 mm). Oversized balloons can cause perforations. Balloon inflation should not exceed 8–10 atm. In severely calcified lesions higher pressure can be necessary. In this case an undersized balloon with a shorter length appropriate for the rest-stenotic segment should be chosen for inflation up to 16–18 atm. However, in rare cases only a cutting balloon (Boston Scientific) is successful *(Figure 10)*.

Inflation time should last at least 30 s and up to 2 min. If the result is unsatisfactory, a second balloon dilatation should always be attempted before stenting is performed. Especially if major dissection occurs, a prolonged dilatation with lower pressure for up to 5 min should be attempted for better alignment of the dissection membrane to the vessel wall.

Balloon dilatation can be very painful, if recanalization occurred in the subintimal space. Deflation and a second start of the dilatation process with slower inflation can reduce the discomfort.

In very tight stenoses or occlusions, passage of the lesion with the balloon can be difficult. A low-profile balloon (Submarine, Invatec) or predilatation with a coronary balloon is recommended in this case. Furthermore, in acute or subacute occlusions, the use of a low-profile balloon can reduce the risk of distal embolization.

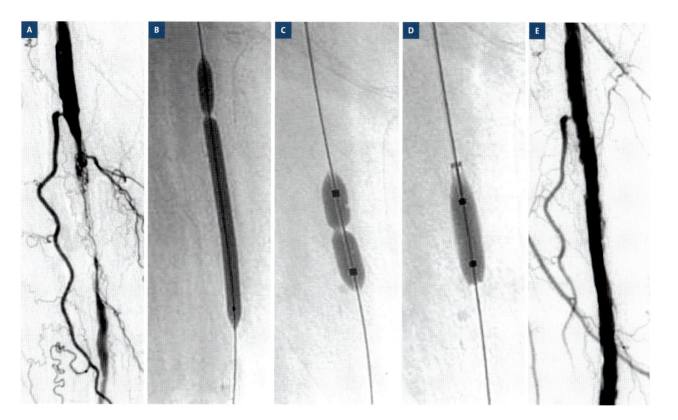

Patency after Balloon Angioplasty

Endovascular balloon angioplasty is well accepted for short segmental disease of the SFA. A guideline for management of peripheral arterial disease, published by the TransAtlantic Inter-Society Consensus Working Group, recommends PTA as first-choice therapy in lesions up to 3 cm in length, whereas occlusions > 5 cm in length should undergo bypass operation. In fact, the reported long-term patencies after balloon angioplasty of SFA lesions are inconsistent, varying from 73% after 4 years to only 23% for long lesions after only 6 months. Besides the length of the lesion, probably also other factors have an influence on long-term outcome, like lesion type (stenosis vs. occlusion), clinical stage (claudication vs. critical ischemia) or outflow.

FIGURES 10A TO 10E.
a) Total occlusion of the right superficial femoral artery.
b) 5/80-mm balloon with 12 atm leaving a short residual stenosis.
c) A shorter balloon (5/20 mm) inflated with 18 atm does not open the stenosis.
d) A 5/10-mm cutting balloon is successful with 8 atm.
e) Final result.

Excimer Laser Recanalization of Superficial Femoral Artery Lesions

Laser Physics

In the early 1980s it could be shown that the majority of laser wavelengths of the electromagnetic spectrum can debulk arteriosclerotic material. For all laser systems, most of the light energy absorbed by the tissue is converted to heat almost instantly. Continuous wave laser, such as the "hot tip" laser used initially for vessel recanalization, induced tissue vaporization by a process of desiccation, coagulation, carbonization and subsequent vaporization. Particularly when the recanalization speed was < 1.5 mm/s, considerable transverse temperature rise was observed and thermal damage to adjacent tissue structures could hardly be avoided. The increase of the vessel-surrounding temperature to 400–500 °C could be deleterious with regard to the long-term results of those interventions. Furthermore, because heavily calcified material is refractory to the ablation mechanism of thermal systems, a recanalization stop due to calcified obstacle causes an unacceptable high risk of perforation.

In contrast to the vaporization with continuous wave lasers, the excimer laser is a pulsed system with extremely short pulse duration, which induces an effect termed optical breakdown or photoablation during a so-called athermic process. The medical systems introduced for angioplasty use xenon chloride 308-nm excimer lasers as the source of energy. At very high energy densities with an extremely short tissue interaction time and extremely high temperature, rise of the irradiated volume provokes a local very fast micro explosion. Thermal damage induced by the excimer laser is minimal, since the pulse duration is much shorter than it takes for the heat to diffuse away from the tip of the catheter.

Excimer Laser-Assisted Recanalization Technique

For laser-assisted SFA recanalization the crossover approach is recommended as for other recanalization techniques. The multifiber excimer laser catheter (7 F or 8 F) is placed at the origin of the occlusion and the activated catheter is advanced the first few millimeters into the occlusion without wire guidance. For further recanalization of the occluded vessel segment either a "step-by-step technique" can be used (for details see Chapter 4) or lasering is performed after passage of the occlu-

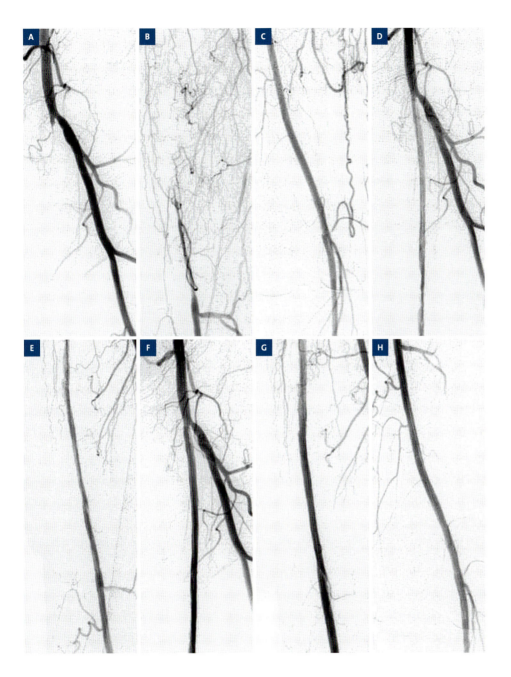

Figures 11a to 11h.
a–c) 20 cm long total occlusion of the left superficial femoral artery.
d, e) After three passes with a 7-F excimer laser.
f–h) Final result after additional balloon dilatation.

sion with the guide wire. Fluoroscopic "road mapping" is used throughout the intervention to verify the alignment of guide wires and catheters to the vessel lumen. Particular attention is given to thoroughly flushing the vessel with saline before lasering to remove remaining contrast medium, as the interaction of laser energy with the contrast medium can produce shock waves, which may result in disruption of the vessel wall with local and distal dissections. If the initial laser passage is performed using a 0.035" hydrophilic guide wire, it is changed for a 0.018" guide wire to allow distal saline flushing during a second or third laser passage of the obstructed area. Finally, the recanalization procedure is completed by complementary balloon dilatations *(Figure 11)*.

Successful recanalization is achieved in > 80% of total SFA occlusion using an excimer laser. With debulking of obstructive material it is possible to transform an occlusion into a stenosis. Subsequently, the final balloon dilatation can be performed with lower pressure, which may reduce arterial wall stress and the rate of subsequent dissections. This may lead to a reduced need for stenting and a reduced stimulation of the mechanisms of restenosis.

Stenting of the Superficial Femoral Artery

The primary success rate for recanalization even of extensive chronic occlusions of the SFA is very high. The most challenging aspect of endovascular therapy is now to maintain patency. Based on the experience in iliac arteries, stents were also advocated to improve patency of the femoropopliteal tract. But, considering the few trials, which are published to date, the use of stents in the SFA is unsatisfactory. However, it has to be kept in mind that the experience is mainly limited to the use of balloon-expandable stents and self-expanding stainless-steel stents. Most important disadvantage of balloon-expandable stents is the deformability by extrinsic compression, which can lead to restenosis and reocclusion in the femoropopliteal tract. By contrast, self-expanding stents show complete recoil after external deformation. Therefore, self-expanding stents should be used in the SFA, an artery, which is subjected to compression, elongation, shortening, and distortion over the whole length. The stainless-steel Wallstent (Meditech, Boston Scientific, Boston, MA, USA), was the first self-expanding stent used in the

SFA. Most important disadvantage of this stent is its significant and unpredictable foreshortening of up to one third of its unconstrained state, making an exact placement difficult (*Figure 12*). Furthermore, the radial force, which is still effective after deployment, may provoke a further enlargement with consequent ongoing foreshortening and development of gaps between initially overlapping stents.

Another concept of self-expansion uses the thermal memory characteristics of nitinol, an elastic intermetallic alloy of nickel and titanium. Preshaped at high temperature to its nominal dimension, the stent is soft and deformable after cooling. When exposed to body temperature during deployment, the stent tends to expand rapidly to its nominal diameter. One of the most distinguishing advantages over the Wallstent is its negligible foreshortening of approximately 5%, making the implantation significantly more precise. Due to the segmental design of most of the nitinol stents (except the spiral stents), the accommodation to the different diameters of the artery is potentially superior compared to the Wallstent.

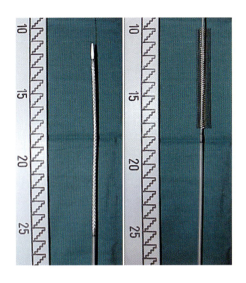

FIGURE 12. *Wallstent before and after release.*

In a multicenter study promising improvements of the long-term patency using nitinol stents in the treatment of long diffuse SFA lesions could be observed. In a sample of 329 SFA procedures stainless-steel Wallstents were used in 166 interventions and nitinol stents in 163 procedures. The mean lesion length was 20 cm and 80% of these lesions were total occlusions. The 1-year primary, assisted primary, and secondary patency rates were 61%, 75%, and 79% for nitinol stents compared to 30%, 53%, and 64% for Wallstents, respectively *(Figure 13)*. Achieving long-term secondary patency of about 80% using nitinol stents in long lesions demonstrates, that this technology is safe, clinically very effective and comparable with results after bypass surgery.

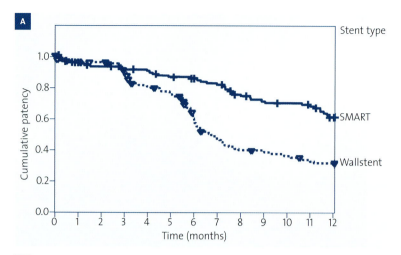

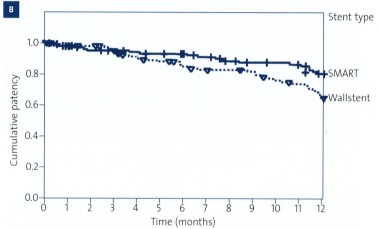

Figures 13a and 13b.
Comparison of the 1-year patency of nitinol stents (SMART) with Wallstents.
a) Primary patency.
b) Secondary patency.

Tips and Tricks

■ Nitinol stents have become the mainstay in the femoropopliteal tract. Balloon-premounted stents should be restricted to short, very calcified stenoses showing significant recoil after balloon angioplasty.

Radiopacy of the nitinol stents is inferior compared to stainless-steel stents, but this fact may only play a role in pelvic and not in femoropopliteal arteries, where overlying tissue is negligible. Some vendors have overcome this drawback by using markers at both ends of the stent. *Table 1* gives an overview of some of the available nitinol stents for the use in the femoropopliteal tract.

Recanalization of the Femoropopliteal Tract

Table 1.

Stent type	Diameter (mm)	Length (mm)	Minimum sheath size (F)	Working length (cm)	Vendor
S.M.A.R.T.™ Control™	6–14	20–100	6–7	80/120	Cordis
Xceed™	5–8	20–120	>6	80/120	Abbott
Absolute™	5–10	28–100	6	80/120	Guidant
Luminexx®	4–14	20–120	6	135	Bard
Conformexx®	6–8	40–120	6	135	Bard
Protégé™	6–9	20–150	6–7	135	ev3
Sentinol™	5–10	20–80	6	75/135	Boston Scientific
Aurora	6–10	20–80	6–7	75/120	Medtronic
Zilver™	6–10	40–80	5–6	80/125	Cook
ASpire™	6–12	25–100	8	50/100	Vascular ARCHITECTS
Optimed Sinusstent	4–10	10–150	5–7	45/150	Optimed
Maris™	6–12	30–120	6	80/120	Invatec
Astron	7–10	20–80	6	70/120	Biotronik
LifeStent™	6–10	20–90	6	75/120	Edwards

Table 1. *Different nitinol stents for use in the femoropopliteal tract.*

Indications for Stenting the Femoropopliteal Artery

Stenting of the SFA remains controversial. Up to now accepted indications for stenting are limited to suboptimal angioplasty results like flow-limiting dissections, especially spiral dissections *(Figure 14)*, a residual pressure gradient >15 mmHg or a remaining stenosis >30% *(Figure 15)*, an elastic recoil as well as failure to maintain initial patency.

The clinical situation should possibly influence the decision for stenting as well. In a recent meta-analysis of long-term results after angioplasty of femoropopliteal lesions collected from 19 studies, the outcomes of 923 balloon dilatations and 473 stent implantations were compared. The 3-year patency rate

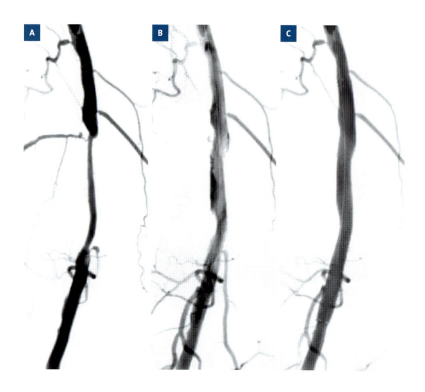

FIGURES 14A TO 14C.
a) Stenosis of the right superficial femoral artery.
b) Major spiral dissection.
c) Final result after stenting.

When dilating long SFA segments, the placement of a stent can substantially improve the aesthetic appearance. In consequence, the luminal diameters proximal and distal to the stent may appear unsatisfactory, inducing the so-called oculostenotic reflex to continue stenting until the entire vessel is covered. This scenario might carry a high risk of restenosis.

Technique of Stent Implantation

After balloon angioplasty, an appropriately sized stent has to be chosen. The stent should cover the whole lesion, and preferably extend for some millimeters into the healthy vessel. Since collaterals almost always have their origin where occlusions start and end, stents have to be placed regardless of these vessels. The occlusion of side branches after stenting is rare. The diameter of self-expanding nitinol stents should be 1–2 mm larger than the reference vessel. Therefore, stents for the SFA will usually have a nominal diameter of 6–7 mm. Postdilatation for adaptation of the stent can be performed with a 6-mm balloon in a 5-mm vessel without the risk of rupture.

after balloon angioplasty was 61% for stenoses and claudication, 43% for stenoses and critical limb ischemia, and 30% for occlusions and critical limb ischemia. The 3-year patency rates after stent implantation were 63–66% and were independent of the clinical state and lesion type.

Recently, Schillinger et al. conducted a randomized monocentric trial including 104 patients with intermittent claudication due to long SFA lesions, where a clear benefit for primary stenting compared to balloon angioplasty and optional stenting in terms of patency and 1-year clinical improvement was demonstrated.

> **TIPS AND TRICKS**
>
> ▪ Indication for stenting is an unsatisfactory angioplasty result.

Recanalization of the Femoropopliteal Tract

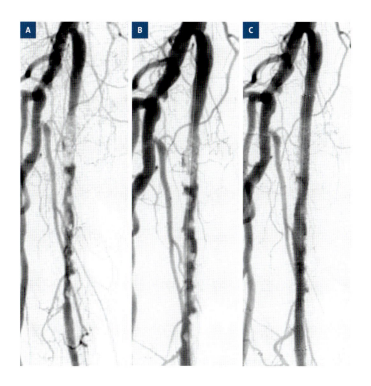

FIGURES 15A TO 15C.
a) Subtotal diffuse occlusion of a highly calcified right superficial femoral artery.
b) Restenoses > 50% after balloon angioplasty.
c) Final result after stenting.

In lesions of the proximal SFA near the origin of the profunda artery the use of balloon-expandable stents for accurate placement seems to be appropriate. However, self-expanding stents can be placed very precisely as well using the following technique: the delivery system of the stent is first placed a few millimeters distal to the intended region.

After the first struts are fully expanded, the stent is pulled to the correct level. During deployment nitinol stents tend to move forward. However, if traction on the delivery system is maintained during the whole release process, precise positioning is also possible with these stents.

> **TIPS AND TRICKS**
>
> ▪ *Nitinol stents for the use in the femoropopliteal tract should be oversized by 1–2 mm.*

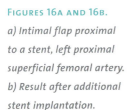

FIGURES 16A AND 16B.

a) Intimal flap proximal to a stent, left proximal superficial femoral artery. b) Result after additional stent implantation.

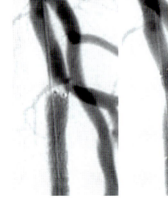

Surveillance after Stenting the Superficial Femoral Artery

Short-Term Follow-Up

Acute occlusion after stenting the SFA, which used to occur more frequently in long lesions, has become a rare complication since technical improvements like the crossover approach, nitinol stents and low-molecular-weight heparin (LMH) have been introduced. The occurrence can be reduced far below 1% using a postinterventional anticoagulation regimen including acetylsalicylic acid (ASA, 100 mg/d), clopidogrel (75 mg/d) and LMH for several days or weeks. Yet, acute thrombosis can be observed despite sufficient anticoagulation, and can be due to a dissection, appearing as a flap immediately adjacent to the proximal end of the stent *(Figure 16)*. In this case, the treatment should be a prolonged balloon dilatation or placement of an additional stent.

Long-Term Follow-Up

Late restenosis or reocclusion by intimal hyperplasia or progressive arteriosclerosis is still a relevant problem in this arterial segment. Restenosis can also continue to emerge even after years. Therefore, periodical follow-up examinations also beyond the time limit of 6 months to 1 year are of highest importance and duplex sonography is the method of choice. We recommend a routine surveillance every 3 months during the first year and twice yearly thereafter. Early reintervention should be performed before reocclusion occurs.

Treatment of In-Stent Restenosis

At the moment, the best technique for treatment of significant in-stent restenosis is balloon angioplasty, which has resulted in acceptable secondary patency rates *(Figure 13b)*. Laser is another potent tool for recanalization of in-stent restenosis or reocclusions. Endovascular atherectomy systems have been used, but published results were discouraging. A recently introduced

TIPS AND TRICKS

- *Close and indefinite surveillance after SFA stenting is mandatory.*

novel atherectomy device (Silverhawk, Fox Hollow, Redwood City, CA, USA) might yield different results. Cutting balloons (Boston Scientific) are available in a maximal length of 2 cm and are therefore only appropriate for focal restenosis. In-stent stenting for dissections, residual stenoses or for lesions at sites of stent fracture is possible, safe, and effective *(Figure 17)*.

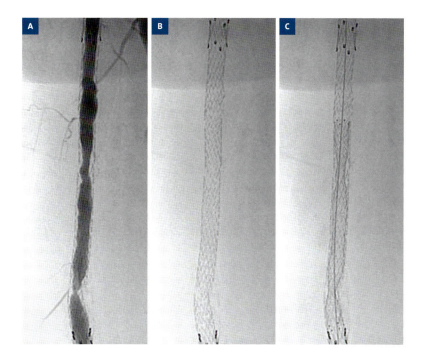

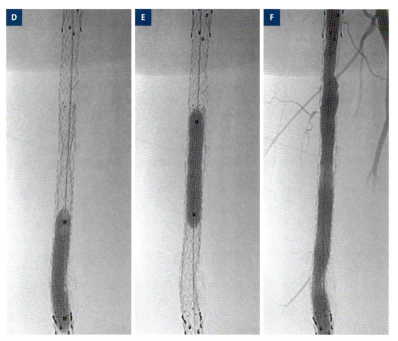

Figures 17a to 17f.
a) In-stent restenosis, left superficial femoral artery.
b) Severe stent fracture at the site of restenosis.
c) In-stent stent implantation.
d, e) Postdilatation.
f) Final result.

Treatment of Acute and Subacute Occlusions of the Superficial Femoral Artery

An embolic or thrombotic occlusion of the femoropopliteal tract often leads to an acute onset of severe symptoms, making an immediate treatment mandatory. Surgical removal of the thrombotic material by a Fogarty catheter in this region can be unsatisfactory due to concomitant atherosclerotic lesions and may lead to distal embolization. Endovascular techniques like thrombus aspiration, thrombolysis, mechanical thrombectomy (X-Sizer [ev3], Straub-Rotarex® [Straub Medical]) as well as conventional balloon angioplasty and stenting or a combination of the techniques are minimally invasive alternatives for these patients.

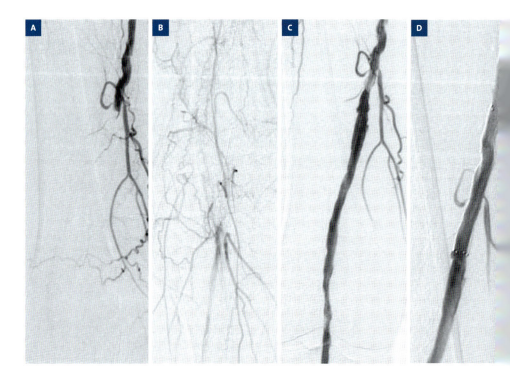

FIGURES 18A TO 18E.

a, b) Acute occlusion of the right distal superficial femoral artery and first segment of the popliteal artery.

c) Result after thrombectomy using the Straub-Rotarex® catheter.

d, e) Final result after additional balloon dilatation and proximal stent implantation.

The first step is to pass the lesion with a 0.018" guide wire, preferably a V18-control-wire (Boston Scientific) to get an impression of the consistency of the occlusion. If no run-off vessels can be visualized, the wire should be brought as far distal as possible supported by a low-profile catheter (e.g., Diver catheter, Invatec, Roncadelle, Italy) or a low-profile balloon (e.g., Submarine balloon, Invatec, Roncadelle, Italy). After retrieval of the wire, gentle contrast injection via the support or balloon catheter and slow retrieval of the catheter can show the level of the reconstitution segment.

In case of a thrombotic occlusion thrombus aspiration can be attempted.

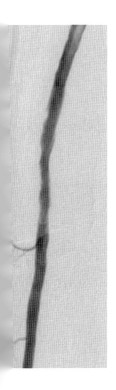

For this purpose larger sheaths (7–9 F), if possible with a detachable hemostatic valve, should be preferred. Then, a 6- to 9-F guiding catheter is gently introduced into the occlusion and aspiration is performed with a 50-ml syringe. In subacute thrombotic or embolic occlusions pretreatment with thrombolytics can prove beneficial.

In longer acute occlusions of the SFA aspiration is often unsuccessful and the use of a thrombectomy device can be recommended as first choice. Various mechanical thrombectomy catheters have been developed using either the vortex principle (e.g., Amplatz thrombectomy catheter [ATD, Microvena], Arrow-Trerotola Thrombolysis System [Arrow]) or utilizing the Bernoulli and Venturi effect for removing the thrombus (e.g., Hydrolyser® [Cordis], Angiojet® [Possis Medical], Oasis® [Boston Scientific]). Many of these devices are successful only in acute thrombotic occlusions and need an additional application of thrombolytic agents in a considerable number of cases.

The Straub-Rotarex® (Straub Medical) combines two essential mechanisms for thrombus recanalization, the mechanical clot fragmentation and removal of the material by continuous negative pressure. It is applicable in acute and also subacute occlusions and does not need additional treatment with thrombolytic agents. A steel spiral coated by an 8-F catheter with two lateral openings at the catheter tip is inserted over a 0.018" guide wire. It is connected to a 40-W electronic motor, which rotates the spiral at a speed of 40,000 rpm additionally generating a continuous vacuum of up to 43 mmHg. Thrombotic material is drawn into the catheter, fragmented by the rotating spiral and transported into a collecting bag at the distal end of the catheter. After recent improvement of the device it can also successfully be used in a crossover approach using an 8-F crossover sheath. Even longer thrombotic occlusions can be recanalized, often without the additional treatment with thrombolytics *(Figure 18)*. However, in case of a severely angulated bifurcation or tortuous pelvic arteries an antegrade approach may be more appropriate to avoid friction of the catheter within the crossover sheath.

Despite the introduction of these thrombectomy catheters, complete removal of the thrombotic material is not possible in a considerable number of patients and local thrombolysis is the next step. Local intraarterial infusion or infiltration of the thrombus using especially designed infusion catheters with side holes (e.g., Cragg-McNamara™ Valved Infusion Catheter, Micro Therapeutics, Inc., Irvine, CA, USA) can be performed in the laboratory or preferably infused over hours or even days using different infusion regimens until a control angiography is performed.

A prerequisite for successful local thrombolysis is to restore a minimal flow by predilatation of the thrombosed segment using an undersized balloon, e.g., a 3/80-mm balloon. Comparison of the efficacy of thrombolytic agents is difficult due to different techniques of local application of the drug and different dosages, however, recent trends lead away from streptokinase and urokinase favoring recombinant tissue plasminogen activator (rtPA). Direct thrombus infiltration using a regimen of 5 mg rtPA given as a bolus followed by a continuous infusion of either 1 mg rtPA + 750 IU heparin/h or 2 mg rtPA + 500 IU heparin/h over a period of 12 and maximally 24–36 h has proven to be highly successful combined with a low complication rate.

> **TIPS AND TRICKS**
>
> ▪ *In acute occlusion of the SFA a combination of mechanical thrombectomy, thrombus aspiration, thrombolysis, balloon angioplasty and stenting should be attempted.*

Recanalization of the Femoropopliteal Tract

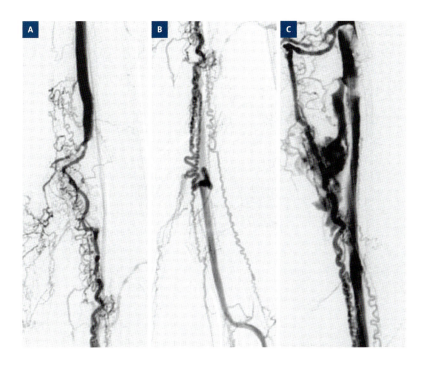
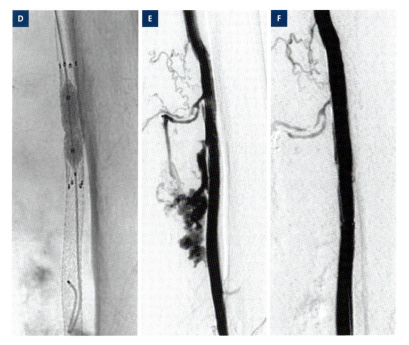

Figures 19a to 19f.

a, b) Calcified occlusion of the distal left superficial femoral artery.
c) Perforation after guide-wire passage through the vessel wall and balloon dilatation.
d) Stent implantation and postdilatation.
e) Ongoing bleeding.
f) Final result after implantation of a covered stent (Fluency 8/40 mm, Bard).

Complications of Recanalization of the Superficial Femoral Artery

Complications after angioplasty of stenoses of the SFA are reported to occur in 0–5% and are nearly exclusively limited to the entry site. The risk of perforation is minimal, if balloons are chosen according to the reference vessel size, which rarely exceeds 5 mm.

In case of perforation and persistent bleeding after passage of the guide wire through the vessel wall during recanalization of total occlusions, a prolonged blockage with a balloon or stenting often leads to a sealing. Nevertheless, a covered stent should be available in the laboratory at any time *(Figure 19)*.

The possibility of peripheral embolization with consequent occlusion of the trifurcation during angioplasty of acute or subacute SFA occlusions has always to be taken into account. Options for treatment are thrombolysis and embolectomy using especially designed devices like the X-sizer. However, most successful is a thrombus aspiration using a larger-sized guiding catheter (6–8 F).

> **TIPS AND TRICKS**
>
> ■ *A covered stent for sealing of perforations should always be available.*

Conclusion

A large number of PAOD patients suffer from claudication due to lesions of the femoropopliteal arteries. Using an appropriate access site and different techniques for recanalization, an endovascular intervention is successful in up to 100% of the cases, even in long and chronic occlusions. Preserving the long-term patency is now the challenge for the interventionalist. If ongoing studies can confirm the first promising results of nitinol stents in the SFA, the still controversially discussed endovascular therapy might be accepted as the first choice therapy for lesions in this arterial segment on a broad basis.

References

1. Becquemin J-P, Favre J-P, Marzelle J, Nemoz C, Corsin C, Leizorovicz A. Systemic versus selective stent placement after superficial femoral artery balloon angioplasty: a multicenter prospective randomized study. J Vasc Surg 2003;37:487–94.

2. Duda SH, Bosiers M, Lammer J, Scheinert D, Zeller T, Tielbeek A, Anderson J, Wiesinger B, Tepe G, Lansky A, Mudde C, Tielemans H, Beregi JP. Sirolimus-eluting versus bare nitinol stent for obstructive superficial femoral artery disease: the SIROCCO II trial. J Vasc Interv Radiol 2005;16:331–8.

3. Gray BH, Sullivan TM, Childs MB, Young JR, Olin JW. High incidence of restenosis/reocclusion of stents in the percutaneous treatment of long-segment superficial femoral artery disease after suboptimal angioplasty. J Vasc Surg 1997;25:74–83.

4. Hayerizadeh BF, Zeller T, Krankenberg H, Scheinert D, Rastan A, Geier S, Braunlich S, Wegscheider K, Biamino G. Long-term outcome of superficial femoral artery stenting using nitinol stents compared with stainless steel stents: a multicenter study. Am J Cardiol 92;2003:Suppl:157.

5. Laxdal E, Jenssen GL, Pedersen G, Aune S. Subintimal angioplasty as a treatment of femoropopliteal artery occlusions. Eur J Vasc Endovasc Surg 2003;25:578–82.

6. Muradin GSR, Bosch JL, Stijnen T, Hunink MGM. Balloon dilation and stent implantation for treatment of femoropopliteal arterial disease: meta-analysis. Radiology 2001;221:137–45.

7. Murray RR, Hewes RC, White RI, Mitchell SE, Auster M, Chang R, Kadir S, Kinnison ML, Kaufman SL. Long-segment femoropopliteal stenoses: is angioplasty a boon or a bust? Radiology 1987;162:473–6.

8. Pemberton M, Nydahl S, Hartshorne T, Naylor AR, Bell PR, London NJ. Colour-coded duplex imaging can safely replace diagnostic arteriography in patients with lower-limb arterial disease. Br J Surg 1996;83:1725–8.

9. Scheinert D, Laird JR, Schroeder M, Steinkamp H, Balzer JO, Biamino G. Excimer laser-assisted recanalization of long chronic superficial femoral artery occlusions. J Endovasc Ther 2001;8:156–66.

10. Schillinger M, Sabeti S, Cejna M, Amighi J, Dick P, Loewe C, Lammer J, Minar E. Balloon angioplasty versus primary stenting in the SFA - a randomized controlled trial. N Engl J Med 2006;354:1879–88.

11. Strecker EP, Gottmann D, Boos IB, Vetter S. Low-molecular-weight heparin (reviparin) reduces the incidence of femoropopliteal in-stent stenosis: preliminary results of an ongoing study. Cardiovasc Intervent Radiol 1998;21:375–9.

12. TASC Working Group TransAtlantic Inter-Society Consensus (TASC). Management of peripheral arterial disease (PAD). J Vasc Surg 2000;31:Suppl:1–296.

Chapter Four

Below-the-Knee Interventions

Introduction

The incidence of peripheral artery obstruction disease (PAOD) is 20% in ages > 65 years and is, therefore, increasing dramatically as the population ages. 30–50% of PAOD patients become symptomatic. 15–30% of patients with lower extremity arterial disease will progress from intermittent claudication to critical limb ischemia (CLI) over the course of their disease. CLI is associated with an extremely poor prognosis: only about half of the patients will be alive without a major amputation 1 year after the onset of CLI (25% will have died and 25% will have required major amputation).

Early reported experience with percutaneous transluminal angioplasty (PTA) of infrapopliteal vessels met with limited success.

Despite recent reports showing primary success rates of > 80–90%, the validity of transcutaneous techniques in patients with stenoses or occlusions in popliteal or infrageniculate arteries is still controversial. The weaknesses of recent nonrandomized studies are, in many cases, the lack of a clear protocol, poorly defined follow-up that does not differentiate between primary, primary assisted and secondary patency rates, and poor documentation of clinical improvement, which is not strictly related to the patency of the treated vessel.

From an interventional perspective, nearly 70% of the arterial lesions are located in the femorotibial tract. Isolated lesions below the knee are present in only 15% of the cases. Approximately 30% of symptomatic PAOD patients have diffuse arterial disease affecting the femoropopliteal tract and the tibial arteries. The majority of CLI patients, most of whom are diabetics, have distal arterial disease with occlusions in the tibial arteries *(Figure 1)*. Despite the presence of combined lesions in the superficial femoral (SFA) and infrapopliteal arteries, it is routine in many interventional centers to treat only the obstructions in the SFA, hoping for an improved runoff through the collateral system. This attitude reflects several factors including technical requirements and limited data on the effectiveness of these procedures in category 3 patients of the Rutherford classification as well as in patients with chronic or subacute

> **Contents DVD**
> 9. PTA of the anterior tibial artery for CLI (11:12 min)
> 10. Multilevel recanalization of left SFA and ATA (10:01 min)

Tips and Tricks

- *The main goals in restoring straight-line, pulsatile flow in ischemic vascular disease are to relieve pain, to allow wound healing, or to regain or maintain ambulatory ability. Long-term primary patency is only a secondary goal in this fragile patient population.*

critical leg ischemia with or without tissue loss (category 4–6) normally considered for surgical bypass or amputation. Particularly patients with lifestyle-limiting claudication are "discriminated". In fact, these patients having a walking capacity of around 50–100 m are often not regarded as adequate surgical candidates because of the mediocre long-term results of femorotibial bypass.

On the other hand, there is not any proven efficacy of a medical therapy and the possibilities of an intensive training program are limited in this patient cohort. The consequence for many patients is to accept a relevant reduction of their functional independence with all negative aspects of a reduced mobility.

The complexity of the problems related to the optimal treatment modality of this patient cohort has to be

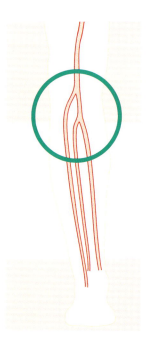
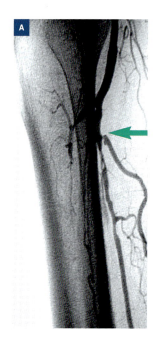
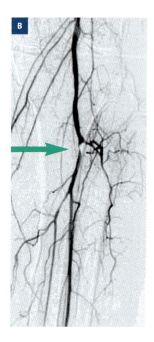

Figures 1a and 1b.
Typical localization and pattern of infragenouidal or tibial lesions.
a) Occlusion of the anterior tibial artery (ATA) and of the fibular artery (AF). Subtotal calcified stenosis of the posterior tibial artery (ATP).
b) Occlusion of the ATA. Subtotal stenosis of the truncus tibiofibularis (TTF).

Patient Evaluation and Diagnosis

reviewed in light of advances in interventional tools and techniques and with the therapy goals in mind.

Technology has improved substantially over the last 5 years with the rapid introduction of new wires, debulking devices, balloons, and stents. Further, endovascular specialists have adopted coronary techniques for interventions in the small infragenicular vessels, resulting in higher rates of technical success. As a result, endovascular intervention has become a first-line therapy in this region.

Nonetheless, in 2006 we do not have any evidence-based guidelines related to the indication for stenting tibial arteries. Furthermore, there are no dedicated stents for infrageniculate application. In case of stenting tibial arteries, coronary, balloon-premounted stents or peripheral self-expandable stents are used.

Patient with chronic obstructions of the popliteal or infrapopliteal arteries present, in the majority of cases, with intermittent claudication. Typically, the patients experience exercise-induced ischemic pain in the calf and foot which resolves within some minutes after discontinuation of walking. Ischemic rest pain or nonhealing ulceration and gangrene occur in about one third of this patient population.

The preinterventional workup includes a clinical examination, standardized treadmill testing for objective measurement of the walking capacity as well as calculation of the Ankle-Brachial Index (ABI) at rest and after exercise.

Color-coded duplex sonography (CCD) is a reliable accurate and reproducible method of determining the exact location and severity of arterial stenoses or occlusions both by direct imaging or by the help of Doppler criteria including the shape of the Doppler spectrum and the peak flow velocity within the stenosis as compared to the reference value.

Despite the dramatic clues showing rest pain, ulcerations or gangrene, also the CLI diagnosis has to be confirmed with objective clinical tests. Alternative causes of foot pain and ulcers, such as Buerger's disease, neurotrophic disease or venous insufficiency, must be excluded.

The typical history with progredient claudication is, in many cases, already a sufficient indication for a correct diagnosis. However, the spectrum of variations and manifestations of CLI is consistent.

Physical examination in suspected CLI should include:
- assessment of elevation pallor (45–60° for 30–60 s),
- dependent rubor,
- venous refill time,
- pulse examination and auscultation for bruits.

Differential Diagnosis Versus Peripheral Neuropathy

Ache, pain, numbness or squeezing sensation, often in the arch of the foot and toes. Severe, sharp, shooting pain that does not necessarily follow the anatomic distribution of nerves may indicate the presence of a neuropathy. Furthermore, dysesthesias, and numbness; temperature sensation can be disturbed in case of neuropathy. Foot becomes shiny, scaly and skeletonized.

Skin coloration can be extremely pale or cyanotic. Usually involves the tips of the toes and the heel of the foot. Ulcers often result from any local trauma. Infections are common.

Pain in PAOD occurs or worsens with reduction of perfusion pressure; most often occurs at night or when patient is in supine position; pain relieved by walking or placing foot in dependent position. Patients who keep their legs in a dependent position for comfort often present with edema of the foot and ankles. Severe pain often precedes the formation of ischemic ulcers or gangrene. Paroxysms lasting minutes to hours both with constant diffuse pain remaining in between. Cold sensations during paroxysms, which suddenly become intolerably hot afterwards. Patients cannot tolerate any physical compression of the leg. Even the weight of bedclothes can cause too much pain. May be obscured by ankle and foot edema. CLI is commonly confused with ischemic neuropathy in patients with diabetes who suffer neurotic pain at early stages of their neuropathy.

Goal of Revascularization for Critical Limb Ischemia

The primary procedural goal is to restore straight-line blood flow to the foot; the clinical goal is to induce healing of skin lesions, to relieve pain, and to avoid major amputation. The primary goal of successful revascularization is, in consequence, not necessarily to achieve long-term patency in the CLI patient population.

When selecting a therapy, the global risk of the procedure versus the limb salvage benefit must be weighed carefully. The potential longer durability associated with surgical bypass must be weighed against the lower-risk, minimally invasive, and repeatable endovascular approach.

Bypass Surgery

The premise that surgery offers better durability than endovascular intervention is based on an analysis of pooled data from multiple nonrandomized studies prior to 1999. When these data are analyzed, the range of reported patency rates is not impressive.

Hunink et al. analyzed the results of femoropopliteal interventions from 26 selected studies published after 1985 involving 4,800 PTA procedures and 4,511 surgical bypasses.

Pooled data from a subset of CLI patients treated with a venous conduit showed a 5-year patency of 66%. The durability of bypass using a synthetic graft in CLI patients was even lower with a 5-year patency of only 47%.

A sample of published results of femoropopliteal and femorotibial bypass grafts (irrespective of disease severity) reveals 1-year patency rates ranging from 33–92% and 5-year patency rates ranging from 38–80%.

Primary and secondary patency rates associated with surgery tend to lag behind limb salvage rates in many published series. This indicates that surgical bypass for CLI, like endovascular procedures, is a "temporary" bypass to support wound healing. The major limitations of surgical therapy are the nonrepeatable use of the veins, procedural morbidity and mortality, and the possibility of limb risk with graft failure.

Interventional Revascularization

> **TIPS AND TRICKS**
>
> ■ *Endovascular therapy should be considered before surgery because it is associated with a lower morbidity and mortality risk.*

Endovascular Intervention

With recent technological advances, such as the new wires, the low-profile balloons, excimer laser and stents, and with the greater interventional experience, more diffuse and distal disease can be treated in the interventional suite.

Single- and multicenter studies and reports published since 1999 show technical success rates > 82% and as high as 98% with limb salvage rates > 85%. These results are equal to or better than individual surgical reports.

Since the clinical benefit of treating CLI is preservation of ambulatory function, long-term patency of treated vessels takes secondary importance behind the primary goal of limb salvage.

The primary reason for the widespread adoption of endovascular intervention in CLI is based on the concept of repeatable recanalization with low complication rates and on the fact, that the surgical option remains open in the majority of the cases after PTA procedures.

Access Methods

A key issue in the successful completion of a complex endovascular intervention is selection of the appropriate vascular access. Two standard approaches are available for femoral, popliteal and tibial artery interventions: the crossover and the antegrade approach.

Crossover Access

The crossover approach from the common femoral artery (CFA) is considered nowadays, in many centers, the standard access technique for femoropopliteal interventions. As compared to the antegrade approach, the technically easy crossover approach is associated with a markedly lower complication rate.

Subsequent navigation of the crossover wire is usually uncomplicated, and the arterial compression bandage typically used to achieve postinterventional hemostasis is applied to the contralateral leg. Thus, the postinterventional flow in the recanalized segment will not be affected, which may contribute to lowering the rate of early thrombotic reocclusions.

To provide optimal support for the recanalization procedure, the use of a crossover sheath is recommended (see *Figure 2*, Chapter 3, page 47).

For technical details of the crossover access see page 46, Chapter 3.

Antegrade Access

The antegrade approach (Page 47, Chapter 3) can be applied in cases where crossover access is not possible due to difficult anatomy of the pelvic vessels (e.g., previous aortobifemoral bypass, stents in the region of the aortic bifurcation, etc.). Some interventionalists prefer the antegrade approach because it provides a more direct access to many lesions in the medial and distal femoropopliteal segment and the infragenouidal arteries, which may be helpful to cross very calcified lesions. It may also allow more precise navigation in the tibioperoneal arteries.

However, when compared to the crossover approach, the antegrade puncture is technically far more challenging, particularly in obese patients. Further, a high puncture of the CFA is usually required to have enough space for navigation of the guide wire into the SFA. Suprainguinal puncture should be avoided due to the high risk of retroperitoneal hemorrhage. Injection of radiocontrast through the needle may help to identify the anatomy of the femoral bifurcation. For this imaging, a slightly lateral projection (25°) should be used to open up the angle of the bifurcation.

For details of antegrade sheath placement see page 47, Chapter 3.

Primary Lesion Crossing

Once the sheath is placed, the target lesion is crossed with a guide wire. Below the knee only atraumatic 0.018" or 0.014" guide wires should be used for this purpose.

Whereas 0.014" guide wires are typically used for stenotic lesions, the preferred guide wire in total occlusions is the V18-control-wire (Boston Scientific Corporation). The high steerability and torqueability of this guide wire permit the operator to drill it through the occlusions in the majority of cases. In some patients with total occlusions of the popliteal artery, the use of a 0.035" hydrophilic guide wire may be necessary to cross the lesion. However, after the initial passage of the occlusion, the 0.035" wire should be exchanged for a less traumatic wire.

The use of guide wire support catheters (Quick-Cross support catheter, Spectranetics, Colorado Springs, or Diver support catheter, Invatec, Roncadelle) can also facilitate wire crossing.

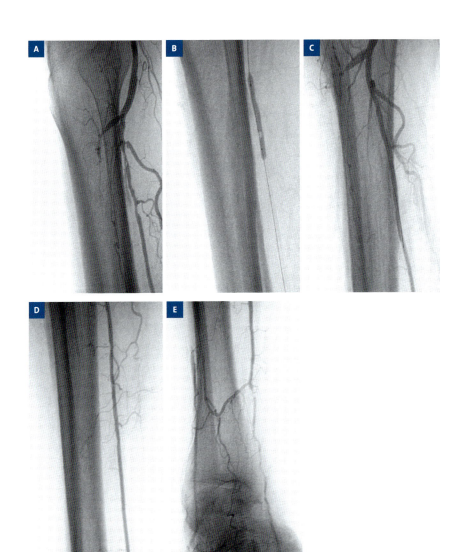

FIGURES 2A TO 2E.

72-year-old female, hypertension, diabetes mellitus for 20 years.

a) Occlusion of the ATA and the AF. The subtotal stenosis of the ATP could only be identified in an oblique protection.

b) After passage of the relevant lesion with a 0.014" guide wire in crossover technique dilatation of the lesion with a 3.5-mm/20-mm low-profile balloon (Amphirion Deep™, Invatec) with 12 bar for 60 s.

c–e) Optimal acute angiographic result. Note the improved runoff with collateral connection to the distal AF and ATA.

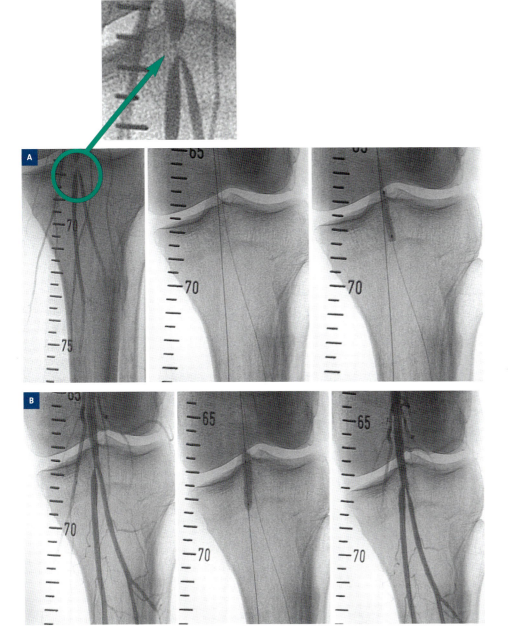

Figures 3a and 3b.

54-year-old male, heavy smoker, claudication 150 m.
a) Atypical high origin of the tibial arteries with functional occlusion of the distal popliteal artery and of the origin of the ATA.
b) After passing the lesion with two 0.014" guide wires (ATA and ATP) alternate dilatation of the obstruction with a 3.0-mm/20-mm coronary balloon. Good angiographic result. Dilatation of the obstruction with a 3.0-mm/20-mm coronary balloon.
Good angiographic result.

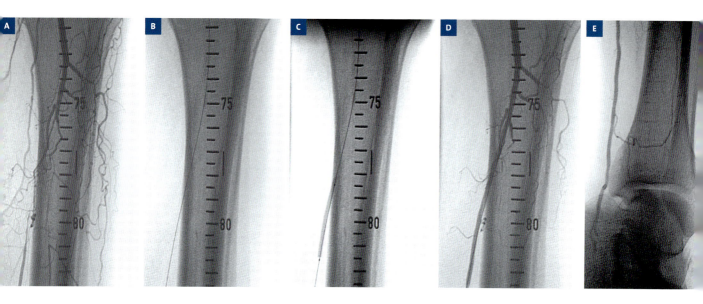

FIGURES 4A TO 4E.
67-year-old, diabetic female, Rutherford 4.
a) The selective angiogram shows a complete occlusion of the ATA and peroneal artery.
b) Using a 0.018" control wire (BSC) it was possible to pass the long ATP occlusion and
c) to dilate the vessel (Submarine Plus™, Invatec, 2.5 mm/40 mm).
d, e) The final result shows a good flow to the foot followed by immediate relief of the rest pain.

Dilatation Process

Only low-profile balloon catheters, preferably with hydrophilic coating (e.g., Submarine Plus™, Invatec), should be used to dilate infrapopliteal vessels, which, in diameter, are very similar to coronary arteries. New coronary-like balloons accepting a 0.014" guide wire (Amphirion Deep™, Invatec) have been developed *(Figure 2)*. It is advisable to use a 90 cm long introducer or to place a 6-F multipurpose guiding catheter through the crossover sheath with the tip in the distal SFA or popliteal artery. In this way the support for the subsequent lesion crossing with the balloon catheter is enhanced and a delivery of stents to the infrapopliteal arteries is protected. Dimensions of the PTA balloon should be chosen according to the proximal and distal reference segment (diameter ranges from 2.5–4 mm) *(Figure 3, 4)*.

> **TIPS AND TRICKS**
>
> ■ *Oversizing should be avoided to reduce the risk of dissections in these fragile vessels.*

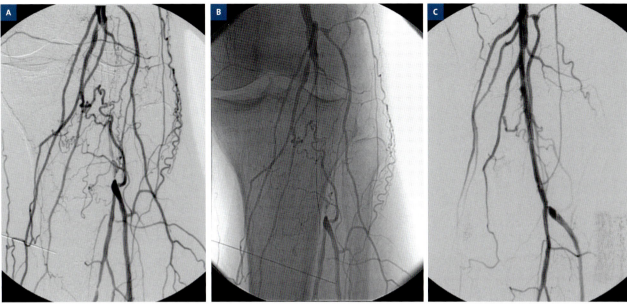

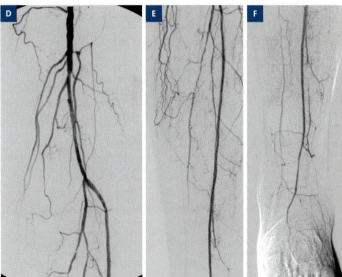

FIGURES 5A TO 5F.

56-year-old male, heavy smoker, Rutherford 3 with an ABI = 0.55 and a walking capacity < 100 m.

a) The selective angiogram shows an occlusion of the PA up to the origin of the ATA. Distal occlusion of the ATP, small AF.

b) The first attempt to wire the occlusion shows an incorrect subintimal position of the tip of the V18 guide wire (BSC).

c) After redirection of the guide wire and using a 2.2-mm excimer laser catheter (Spectranetics) a recanalization of the occlusion could be achieved.

d–f) After three laser passes the intervention could be concluded as stand-alone procedure with a straight-line flow via ATA.

Excimer Laser Recanalization of Total Occlusions: the Step-by-Step Technique

One limitation of conventional recanalization techniques remains the partial inability to cross total occlusions. As an alternate method of recanalization, laser ablation can be used in a step-by-step manner where the guide wire and then a laser catheter are sequentially advanced and activated (millimeter by millimeter) until the occlusion or stenosis is crossed (see *Figure 5*).

In a first step the guide wire is advanced into the origin of the occlusion over which the appropriately sized excimer laser catheter is advanced until the tip is at the occlusion origin.

In a second step the excimer laser catheter is advanced into the first few millimeters of the occlusion without wire guidance. For further recanalization of the occluded vessel segment, the activated laser catheter is advanced stepwise for a short (< 5 mm) distance without wire guidance, followed by further crossing with the guide wire in a step-by-step technique.

The advancement of the activated laser catheter must be performed very slowly, not exceeding 1 mm/s. To enter the patent distal segment of the artery, it is recommended to cross the last segment of the occlusion with the guide wire alone (angled or straight tip) before lasing.

Particular care should be taken to avoid vessel wall dissections distal to the original occlusions.

Excimer Laser Debulking Technique

After the wire has crossed the lesion, with or without the aid of the excimer laser step-by-step technique, the recanalization of the atheroma and/or the thrombus is achieved with multiple passes of an appropriately sized laser catheter. The excimer laser's ability to remove atheroma and thrombus provides the progressive simplification of a complex, diffuse lesion or occlusion into a focal stenosis that is easily treated by balloon angioplasty *(Figure 6)*.

The debulking process of the excimer laser is partially comparable with an open atherectomy.

> **TIPS AND TRICKS**
>
> ▪ *Note: Advancing the laser catheter through moderately calcified lesions may require more pulses of laser energy than fibrous atherosclerotic tissue.*

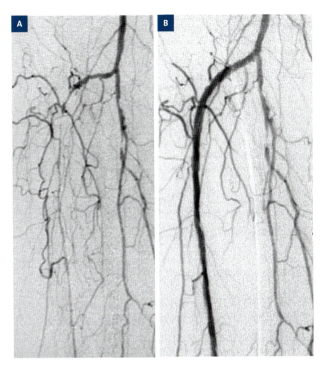

FIGURES 6A AND 6B.
a) Complete obstruction of all tibial arteries. Only the distal segment of ATA is detectable. After excimer laser-assisted debulking and passage with a 0.018" guide wire a dilatation with a low-profile balloon (Submarine Plus™, Invatec, 3 mm/40 mm) could be performed.

b) After repeated balloon inflations optimal angiographic result with clearly improved runoff. The 69-year-old male, diabetic patient had an ulceration at the calcaneus, healing within 3 months postintervention and permitting to put on shoes after nearly 2 years and to walk > 200 m.

Optimization of Final Result

TIPS AND TRICKS

- *Improving the ablation effectivity: While the laser catheter is activated, infuse saline or lactated Ringer's solution.*
- *Expel any residual contrast from the sheath or guiding catheter or the inner channel of the laser catheter.*
- *Under fluoroscopy, confirm that the tip of the laser catheter is in contact with the lesion but do not inject contrast.*

Advancing the catheter faster than 1 mm/s may result in dottering with the potential to cause distal embolization or dissections.

Repeat as many laser trains as necessary to cross and debulk the lesion.

Saline Infusion Technique

Saline can be administered through the sheath (antegrade approach) or laser catheter inner lumen (contralateral approach). When the contralateral approach is used, 0.018" or 0.014" guide wires have to be chosen allowing an adequate saline infusion at the treatment site via y-connector.

The final result of the angioplasty should be evaluated and confirmed using selective angiographic imaging (*Figure 7*).

In case of major, flow-limiting dissections that cannot be controlled by prolonged balloon inflations, stent implantation should be considered to achieve an acceptable hemodynamic result. Coronary stents are useful in infrapopliteal vessels with an average vessel diameter ranging from 2.5–4.0 mm. Balloon-expandable stents should be considered for lesions of the tibio-peroneal arteries. Self-expanding stents should be considered for more proximal vessel segments, including the tibio-peroneal trunk and the popliteal artery.

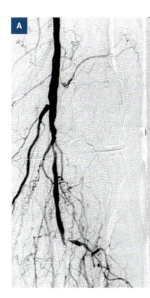
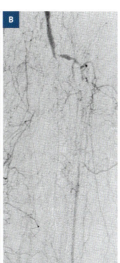
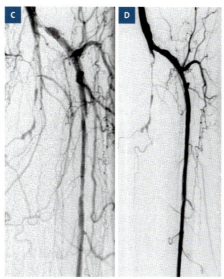

Figures 7a to 7d.

68-year-old male, Rutherford 5, diabetes mellitus, renal failure.
a, b) Complete occlusion of all tibial arteries with minimal perfusion of the distal ATA.
c) After two passes with a 2.2-mm excimer laser catheter (Spectranetics) a good blood flow could be restored.
d) Repeat inflations with a low-profile balloon (Submarine Plus™, Invatec, 3.5 mm/40 mm) could seal the partial dissections with a good final angiographic result.

Managing Procedural Complications

Although infrequent, procedural complications do occur in complex infrapopliteal or tibioperoneal interventions.

Spasm
- Nitroglycerin (0.2–0.6 mg intra-arterially),
- prolonged balloon inflation,
- stent.

Major Dissection
- Prolonged balloon inflation,
- stent.

Local Thrombus
- Local lytic administration (3–8 mg rtPA [recombinant tissue plasminogen activator]),
- abciximab,
- mechanical thrombolysis,
- laser.

Distal Embolization
- Mechanical thrombolysis,
- local lytic administration,
- abciximab,
- laser (with 0.9-mm catheter for distal vessels).

Perforation
- Prolonged balloon inflation,
- stent,
- endovascular prosthesis.

Tips and Tricks

- Within the large number of reports on revascularization techniques for the treatment of CLI, there is no definitive data that universally supports one treatment strategy over the others.

Postprocedural Treatment

During the intervention, 5000 IU heparin should be administered intra-arterially. Anticoagulation may be continued for 24 h (1,000–1,200 IU/h heparin intravenously) with an activated partial thromboplastin time of 60–80 s. In case of recanalization of total occlusions or stent implantation we recommend to prolong the anticoagulation with weight-adjusted low-molecular heparin for 3 weeks.

Acetylsalicylic acid (100 mg/d) is given to all patients.

Clopidogrel (75 mg/d) is prescribed to patients who received stents for at least 6 weeks. In selected cases, particularly after administration of drug-eluting stents a longer duration of clopidogrel administration may be considered.

We have to stress the fact that these are personal recommendations not supported by scientific data, but only by the daily clinical experience.

Postinterventional Surveillance and Patient Follow-Up

Patients with CLI require lifelong follow-up.

Patients with nonhealing ulcers or minor amputations require rehabilitation after their revascularization procedure to ensure their return to an ambulatory status.

Although the primary goal is wound healing and limb salvage, patency of the treated arterial segment can be preserved through surveillance programs that identify flow-limiting restenosis before complete occlusion of the conduit vessel.

Rigorous surveillance may also have an impact on long-term survival.

> **TIPS AND TRICKS**
>
> ■ *After successful revascularization, aggressive wound care is essential to ensure rapid healing. The interventionalist treating a CLI patient must develop a basic understanding of wound care procedures and refer the patient to the proper specialist for further care.*
> ■ *After an endovascular intervention a multidisciplinary approach, including prevention, patient education, endovascular intervention and the comprehensive treatment of foot ulcers, may reduce the amputation rate by 43–85%.*

> **FOLLOW-UP RECOMMENDATION**
>
> 1-, 3-, 6-, 12-month controls, then every 6–12 months, including:
> ■ patient history,
> ■ clinical examination,
> ■ ABI at rest and, if possible, after treadmill test,
> ■ color flow duplex scanning.
>
> If noninvasive tests are abnormal or reocclusion is suspected:
> ■ magnetic resonance angiography or
> ■ intraarterial angiography
> to evaluate patient for endovascular or surgical reintervention.

> **TIPS AND TRICKS**
>
> ■ *The successful management of a patient with CLI is complex and requires the input of multiple medical professionals.*

Because of the high incidence of comorbidities (between 10–30% of CLI patients will have a major nonfatal or fatal cardiovascular event over 6–12 months), all CLI patients should be evaluated regularly for coronary and cerebrovascular involvement.

Further, antiplatelet therapy should be considered for every patient.

Summary of Outcome Results

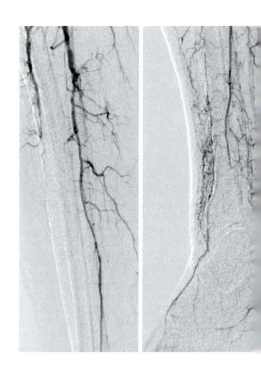

Balloon Angioplasty in Tibial Arteries

Early results of balloon angioplasty for infrapopliteal obstructions showed limited success rates particularly in complex lesions which were mainly related to the limitations of the available interventional material. Based on a series of 60 patients with 72 treated legs and a mean lesion length of 3.8 cm, Soder et al. reported technical success rates of 81% for stenotic and 61% for occlusive infrapopliteal lesions. After a mean follow-up of 10 months a reobstruction rate of 32% for stenotic and 52% for occlusive lesions was recorded.

More recently, refinement of interventional devices (hydrophilic wires and low-profile balloon catheters) led to a substantial improvement of the interventional results. Particularly the availability of long 0.014"- and 0.018"-wire-compatible low-profile balloons (Amphirion Deep™ and Submarine Plus™, Invatec) allows the recanalization of long diffuse lesions with good technical results. Recently, Schmidt et al. reported a technical success rate of 89% in a cohort of 56 patients (82% diabetics) with critical limb ischemia recanalized with low-profile ballons with balloon length of up to 12 cm. The mean lesion length was 18.5 cm. Limb salvage rate was 100% and 72% of patients showed freedom of critical limb ischemia after 3 months (*Figure 8*).

Stenting of Tibial Arteries

Endovascular stenting using balloon-expandable coronary stents has recently been shown to be of potential value to improve the results of infrapopliteal angioplasty for patients with critical limb ischemia and lifestyle-

Below-the-Knee Interventions

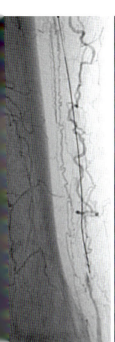
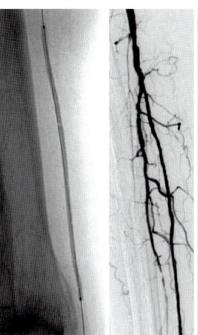
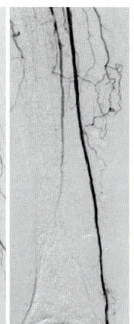
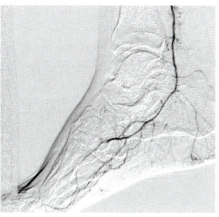

Figures 8a to 8g.
a, b) Long diffuse occlusion of the anterior and posterior tibial artery.
c, d) Recanalization with a hydrophilic steerable 0.018"-wire (Control wire, Boston Scientific) and PTA with a long lower-profile balloon (Submarine Plus™, Invatec).
e-g) Final result with substantially improved blood flow to the foot.

limiting claudication. In a series of 51 patients and 95 lesions which were randomly treated by PTA or stenting Rand et al. could demonstrate a significantly improved patency rate in the stent group of 79.7% vs. 45.6% (p<0.05). Similar observations were made by our group in a series of 112 patients with 132 treated limbs. 74 patients were treated with angioplasty and 58 patients underwent stenting. Overall, significantly better results were observed in the stent group (interventional success 95% vs. 79%; p<0.01; clinical improvement 90% vs. 74%; p<0.05; clinical patency at 12 months 84% vs. 53%; p<0.01) (*Figure 9*).

Drug-Eluting Stents

Nevertheless, according to systematic angiographic follow-up investigations performed in the stent group of the aforementioned investigation, reobstruction rates of coronary bare-metal stents in tibial arteries are exceeding 50% after 12 months. Therefore, the use of drug-eluting stents could be of major benefit for the treatment of patients with tibial artery disease. Within an independent, single-center registry performed at our institution data of 30 patients treated for symptomatic infrapopliteal obstructions with sirolimus-eluting balloon-expandable stents were compared with

> **TIPS AND TRICKS**
>
> ■ *Treatment consists of excimer laser angioplasty + PTA + optional stenting, with the primary endpoints being limb salvage and total survival at 6 months.*

30 patients receiving bare-metal balloon-expandable stents. During follow-up, there were seven unrelated deaths (sirolimus n = 3, bare metal n = 4). The rates of major amputation, bypass surgery or TLR were all 0% for the sirolimus group compared with 10.0%, 0%, and 23.3% in the control group. Angiographic follow-up revealed a significantly reduced in-stent reobstruction rate: stent occlusions 0% vs. 17.4% (p = 0.032), restenosis (>50%) 0% vs. 39.1% (p = 0.0007), confirming that sirolimus-eluting stents are safe and effective for treatment of focal infrapopliteal obstructions.

LACI Trial: Excimer Laser Angioplasty in Critical Limb Ischemia

CLI patients (Rutherford category 4–6) who were poor bypass candidates and who had culprit lesions in the SFA, popliteal and/or infrapopliteal arteries were enrolled in this study.

Poor surgical candidacy was determined if one or more of three conditions were met:
■ no venous conduit was available for creating a bypass;
■ no suitable distal anastamosis site existed;
■ or comorbid conditions placed the patient in American Society of Anesthesiologists (ASA) class 4 or higher.

At 15 sites in the USA and Germany, the LACI Trial enrolled 145 patients with 157 critically ischemic limbs and 423 lesions.

Patient and limb characteristics were typical of patients with systemic vascular disease, with a high incidence of diabetes, hypertension and cardiac disease.

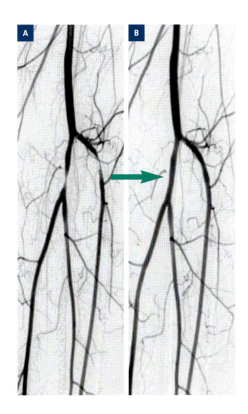

Figures 9a and 9b.
68-year-old male, severe claudication (< 100 m).
a) Restenosis of the TTF and ATA both dilated 6 months earlier.
b) Successful primary stent implantation with excellent result and complete relief of symptoms.

LACI patients presented with severe and diffuse vascular disease typical of CLI.

Of the 423 lesions, 41% were in the SFA, 15% in the popliteal artery, and 41% in infrapopliteal arteries.

Further, 70% of the patients had a combination of stenoses and occlusions, making treatment very complex.

Use of the excimer laser led to an increase in the ability to treat this very complex patient population. Despite a failed guide-wire crossing in 8% of the cases, laser treatment was delivered in 99% of the cases with adjunctive balloon angioplasty successfully performed in 96% of the cases.

In-hospital serious adverse events (SAEs) were extremely low in this very fragile patient group. There were no deaths or surgical interventions as a result of the procedure, and no patient had acute limb ischemia after intervention.

In 45% of the cases included in the LACI Trial a stent was implanted (n = 70, not stented n = 85). Location: 61% SFA, 38% popliteal, and 16% tibial arteries (Laird et al. 2006).

The rate of survival with limb salvage was 93%. Independently of the location, stents improved the acute results significantly. Stenting affected the rate of limb salvage positively (4% vs. 7%).

In this very important trial it has been demonstrated that the use of stents below the knee is safe and effective also recanalizing very complex lesions.

During follow-up, reintervention procedures to reopen symptomatic stenosed or occluded lesions were expected, however, were given only to 16% of patients.

SAEs during the 6-month follow-up period included 10% mortality, almost exclusively from cardiac causes; no patient died within 30 days of the index procedure. Major amputation was required in eleven cases, while four limbs received surgical revascularization.

Comparative Summary of Treatment Options for Critical Limb Ischemia

With 93% the LACI Trial showed that laser-assisted PTA provided a limb salvage rate as high as the reference values observed for a best-case treatment strategy given to patients who were good bypass candidates, while not affecting patient mortality.

LACI achieved limb salvage rates comparable to the "gold standard" of bypass surgery, without higher SAEs.

The clinical advantage of the LACI strategy is that a single intravascular regimen used achieved a lower rate of major amputation in a more extensively diseased population than did PTA in simpler disease patterns. No other interventional technique has been supported with such a large patient population treated in multiple centers.

TIPS AND TRICKS

The LACI Trial demonstrates that excimer laser-assisted endovascular intervention for chronic CLI offers clinical and technical advantages over past endovascular techniques for CLI.

References

1. Ansel GM. Endovascular treatment of femoral and popliteal arterial occlusive disease. J Invasive Cardiol 2000;12:382–8.

2. Ansel GM, George BS, Botti Jr CF, et al. Infrapopliteal endovascular techniques: indications, techniques, and results. Curr Interv Cardiol Rep 2001;3:100–8.

3. Baird RN, Bradley MD, Murphy KP. Tibioperoneal angioplasty and bypass. Acta Chir Belg 2003;103:383–7.

4. Balmer H, Mahler F, Do DD, et al. Angioplasty in chronic critical limb ischemia: factors affecting clinical and angiographic outcome. J Endovasc Ther 2002;9:403–10.

5. Brillu C, Picquest J, Villapadierna F, et al. Percutaneous transluminal angioplasty for management of critical ischemia in arteries below the knee. Ann Vasc Surg 2001;15:175–81.

6. Bull PG, Mendel H, Hold M, et al. Distal popliteal and tibioperoneal transluminal angioplasty: long-term follow-up. J Vasc Interv Radiol 1992;3:45–53.

7. Dorros G, Jaff MR, Dorros AM, Mathiak LM, He T. Tibioperoneal (outflow lesions) angioplasty can be used as primary treatment in 235 patients with critical limb ischemia: five-year follow-up. Circulation 2001;104:2057–62.

8. Faglia E, Mantero M, Caminiti M, et al. Extensive use of peripheral angioplasty, particular infrapopliteal, in the treatment of ischemic diabetic foot ulcers: clinical results of a multicentric study of 221 consecutive diabetic subjects. J Intern Med 2002;252:225–32.

9. Feiring AJ, Wesolowski AA, Lade S. Primary stent-supported angioplasty for treatment of below-knee critical limb ischemia and severe claudication: early and one-year outcomes. J Am Coll Cardiol. 2004;44:2307-14.

10. Gray BH, Laird JR, Ansel GM, et al. Complex endovascular treatment for critical limb ischemia in poor surgical candidates: a pilot study. J Endovasc Ther 2002;9:599–604.

11. Hunink MG, Wong JB, Donaldson MC, Meyerovitz MF, Harrington DP. Patency results of percutaneous and surgical revascularization for femoropopliteal arterial disease. Med Decis Making. 1994;14:71-81.

12. Jamsen T, Manninen H, Tulla H, et. al. The final outcome of primary infrainguinal percutaneous transluminal angioplasty in 100 consecutive patients with chronic critical limb ischemia. J Vasc Interv Radiol 2002;13:455–63.

13. Laird JR, Zeller T, Gray BH, Scheinert D, Vranic M, Reiser C, Biamino G. LACI Investigators. Limb salvage following laser-assisted angioplasty for critical limb ischemia: results of the LACI multicenter trial. J Endovasc Ther. 2006;13:1-11.

14. Matsagas MI, Rivera MA, Tran T, et al. Clinical outcome following infra-inguinal percutaneous transluminal angioplasty for critical limb ischemia. Cardiovasc Intervent Radiol 2003;26:251–5.

15. Rand T, Basile A, Cejna M, Fleischmann D, Funovics M, Gschwendtner M, Haumer M, Von Katzler I, Kettenbach J, Lomoschitz F, Luft C, Minar E, Schneider B, Schoder M, Lammer J. PTA versus carbofilm-coated stents in infrapopliteal arteries: pilot study. Cardiovasc Intervent Radiol. 2006;29:29-38.

16. Scheinert D, Laird JR, Biamino G, et al. Excimer laser-assisted recanalization of long, chronic superficial femoral artery occlusions. J Endovasc Ther 2001;8:156–66.

17. Schmidt A, Bräunlich S, Ulrich M, Scheinert S, Biamino G, Scheinert D. Balloon angioplasty of diffuse infrapopliteal lesions: clinical and angiographical follow-up. Oral presentation at Leipzig Interventional Course(LINC)2006.

18. Schwarten DE, Cutcliff WB. Arterial occlusion disease below the knee: treatment with percutaneous transluminal angioplasty performed with low-profile catheters and steerable guidewires. Radiology 1998;169:71–4.

19. Sivananthan UM, Browne TF, Thorley PJ, et al. Percutaneous transluminal angioplasty of the tibial arteries. Br J Surg 1994;81:1282–5.

20. Soder HK, Manninen HI, Jaakkola P, Matsi PJ, Rasanen HT, Kaukanen E, Loponen P, Soimakallio S. Prospective trial of infrapopliteal artery balloon angioplasty for critical limb ischemia: angiographic and clinical results. J Vasc Interv Radiol. 2000;11:1021-31.

21. Sprayregen S, Sniderman KW, Sos TA, Vieux U, Singer A, Veith FJ. Popliteal artery branches: percutaneous transluminal angioplasty. AJR 1980;135:945–50.

22. Wagner HJ, Rager G. Infrapopliteal angioplasty: a forgotten region. Rofo Fortschr Geb Rontgenstr Neuen Bildgeb Verfahr 1998;168:415–20.

23. Wolfle K, Schaal J, Rittler S, et al. Infrainguinal bypass grafting in patients with end-stage renal disease and critical limb ischemia: is it worthwhile? Zentralbl Chir 2003;128:709–14.

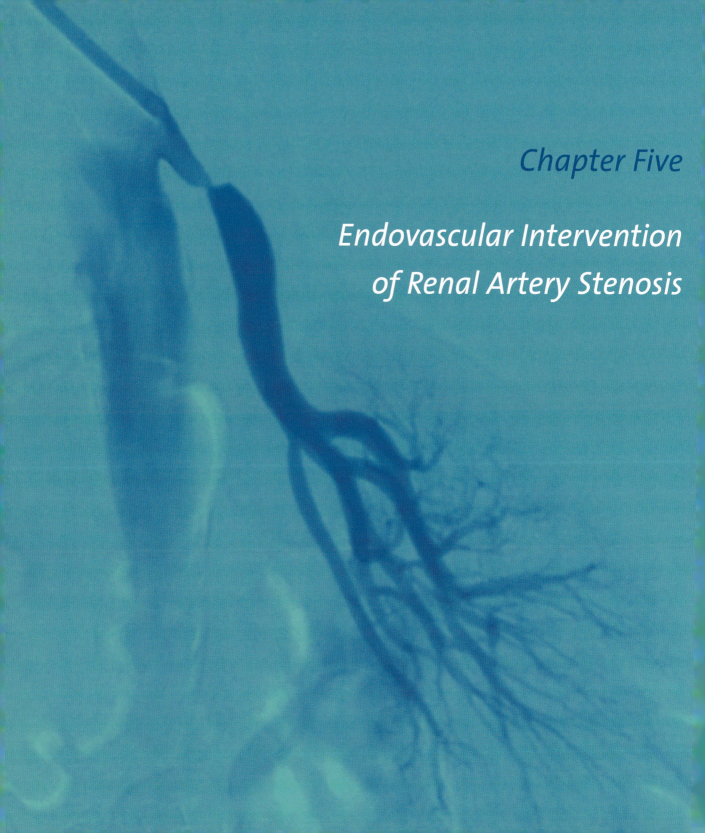

Chapter Five

Endovascular Intervention of Renal Artery Stenosis

Introduction

Aging of our population and technical improvements of screening methods have led to an increase in diagnosis of renovascular disease. With refined equipment, now available for endoluminal treatment of renal artery stenosis (RAS), and evidence for the effectiveness of this therapy, although not derived from randomized trials, renal artery angioplasty is highly accepted for treatment of arterial hypertension, or even more importantly, for improvement or preservation of renal function due to renovascular disease in selected patients.

This article will serve as a brief overview of widely accepted indications, screening methods, and modern technology of renal artery angioplasty.

Contents DVD

11. PTA and stenting of left renal artery (08:05 min)

Diagnostics of Renal Artery Stenosis

The true prevalence of RAS in unselected patients is unknown, and estimates differ greatly according to patient age, clinical presentation and concomitant disease. Newer studies revealed a high prevalence of up to 30% of RAS in patients presenting for angiography with coronary or peripheral artery disease.

Screening

Clinical characteristics might help to increase the probability to diagnose RAS and, thus, increase the effectiveness of further noninvasive screening. Scores for prediction of the existence of RAS include characteristics like drug resistance of arterial hypertension, renal failure due to angiotensin-converting enzyme (ACE) inhibitor treatment, worsening of hypertension within a short period of time, presence of abdominal bruits, elevated serum creatinine concentration, hypokalemia, and presence of generalized atherosclerotic vascular disease.

However, sensitivity and specificity of these scores are not high enough to reliably exclude the existence of RAS in patients with a low probability.

Noninvasive Testing

Algorithms for RAS screening are a matter of ongoing debates. Earlier noninvasive methods such as nuclear renal-flow scanning and plasma renin assays with and without stimulation by ACE blockers are less commonly used, because of a wide range in sensitivity and specificity.

Magnetic resonance angiography (MRA) is noninvasive and does not require iodinated contrast media or ionizing radiation. In addition to measurements of the degree of the stenosis, the size and volume of the kidney can be determined. By using a combination of different techniques, sensitivity and specificity for detection of proximal RAS are as high as 90–100%. Disadvantages of MRA include its high costs, lack of widespread availability, and the need for considerable operator experience in

> **TIPS AND TRICKS**
>
> ■ The reliability of clinical signs of renal artery stenosis is low.

obtaining and interpreting the images. Techniques for grading the hemodynamic effect of RAS by MRA were recently introduced, but have yet to be further evaluated.

Spiral computed tomography (CT) is a reliable tool to image main and accessory renal arteries. Combining different modalities of reconstruction, sensitivity and specificity are around 95%. Fast CT scanners are also able to quantify renal perfusion and segmental renal function, but the impact of this functional information for the workup of patients with RAS, like for MRA, has to be further evaluated. The major disadvantage of CT scanning as a screening test is the high amount of contrast medium in this patient group with often preexisting renal insufficiency.

Color duplex sonography has some features of an ideal screening test in being widely available and inexpensive. However, the results are highly dependent on the investigator's experience, and it is often claimed to be nondiagnostic in a considerable number of patients due to obesity and overlying bowel gas. Yet, intrarenal Doppler signals of segmental renal arteries can be obtained in almost every patient. The Resistive Index (RI), calculated from these signals, can be used for detection of RAS (Table 1).

However, the sensitivities and specificities vary significantly among the reported studies. Besides screening for RAS the RI was recently found to be very useful for prediction of the outcome after interventional treatment. It was found, that an RI with a value of > 0.8 of the contralateral renal segmental arteries was a strong predictor for treatment failure concerning arterial hypertension and renal function. Conversely, a lower RI was associated with improvement in both, renal function and blood pressure after the correction of RAS. In consequence, patients with an RI > 0.8 could be excluded from further diagnostic workup (for more details see Chapter 1). However, these findings are not supported by all investigators and should therefore be confirmed in further, preferably randomized trials.

TABLE 1.

	Relevant stenosis	Pitfalls and shortcoming
Intrastenotic PSV	> 180 cm/s	Precise angle correction difficult to obtain
RI	< 0.45	Rare finding
Side-to-side difference of the RI (ΔRI)	> 5%	No value in bilateral stenosis
Renal/aortic index of PSV	> 3	Precise angle correction is a prerequisite

TABLE 1. *Duplex-sonographic criteria for the detection of renal artery stenosis. PSV: peak systolic velocity; RI: Resistive Index.*

Indications and Patient Selection for Renal Artery Angioplasty

Arterial Hypertension

Reports on the effect of revascularization on blood pressure control have generally been favorable, although complete resolution of hypertension after renal angioplasty is uncommon and confined to the rare group of fibromuscular dysplasia of the renal artery, which accounts for maximally 10% of RAS. In contrast to observational studies, few randomized trials published only recently uniformly demonstrated that renal angioplasty has no significant effect on blood pressure control. The largest of these randomized trials, however, revealed, that patients treated conservatively had to undergo percutaneous transluminal angioplasty (PTA) for uncontrolled blood pressure or deterioration of renal function under antihypertensive therapy in up to 50% during follow-up. Further critical aspects of this study were the inclusion of patients with stenoses of ≥ 50%, which might increase the risk of including patients without hemodynamically significant RAS. And finally, restenosis after PTA was frequently found in this trial during follow-up because of a low rate of stent implantations.

In spite of these trials, there is still a general agreement, that interventional treatment of RAS should not be refused in specific clinical situations like accelerated hypertension (sudden worsening of previously controlled hypertension), refractory hypertension (hypertension resistant to treatment with at least three medications of different classes), and malignant hypertension (hypertension with coexistent evidence of end-organ damage). Especially for patients with "flash" pulmonary edema or patients with unstable angina in the setting of significant RAS, according to observational registries, angioplasty can be highly effective *(Table 2)*. Finally, a meta-analysis of the randomized trials confirmed a moderate, but significant effect of RAS angioplasty on arterial blood pressure.

TABLE 2. *Factors determining the decision pro and contra invasive treatment of renal artery stenosis in hypertensive patients.*
RI: Resistive Index.

TABLE 2.

Pro	Contra
Young patients	Older patients, long-lasting hypertension
Hypertension refractory to triple medication	Easily controlled hypertension
Progressive renal failure under antihypertensive medication	No rise of serum creatinine under antihypertensive medication
RI of nonstenotic kidney < 0.8	RI of nonstenotic kidney ≥ 0.8
Fibromuscular dysplasia	
History of flash pulmonary edema	

Renal Insufficiency

On the basis of registries of patients with end-stage renal failure some authors assume, that renovascular obstructive disease may be the primary causative factor in up to 20% of the cases. There are several reports about the effect of RAS angioplasty on further development of renal function in patients with preexisting renal insufficiency. Improvement of renal function is reported to range from 10% to up to 60% of the cases after angioplasty. The nature of renal dysfunction is progression; therefore, stabilization after revascularization can be regarded as a success. In many studies the majority of patients showed no significant change in kidney function after angioplasty and therefore might be considered stabilized. However, the remaining group of 20–35% of patients developed further rise in serum creatinine, sometimes with a rapid progression to end-stage renal failure and permanent dialysis dependence after angioplasty.

Up to now, there are no reliable guidelines for selecting patients who will recover renal function after revascularization. Patients with high serum creatinine levels are generally considered to have the least chance for improvement. Occasionally, however, these patients have the largest benefit and even recover from permanent dialysis. At least in case of bilateral high-grade stenosis or stenosis of a single organ there is strong evidence, that angioplasty is effective, independent of the baseline serum creatinine level. Other predictive factors for a positive outcome are a short history or progressive deterioration of renal dysfunction and relatively well-preserved renal size. An elevated serum creatinine is indicative of a loss of more

Pro	Contra
Progressive renal failure	Stable renal failure
High-grade stenosis (> 80%) + normal serum creatinine	Unilateral 50–80% stenosis + normal serum creatinine
Unilateral stenosis + slight elevation of serum creatinine	Unilateral stenosis + high serum creatinine
Bilateral stenoses or unilateral stenosis with single kidney independent of serum creatinine	
Unilateral stenosis and markedly lower GFR on affected side	Unilateral stenosis and equal GFR on both sides
Renal length ≥ 8 cm	Renal length < 8 cm
RI of nonstenosed kidney < 0.8	RI of nonstenosed kidney ≥ 0.8

TABLE 3. *Factors for determining the decision pro or contra invasive treatment of renal artery stenosis in terms of benefit for renal function. GFR: glomerular filtration rate; RI: Resistive Index.*

Angiographic Evaluation of Renal Artery Stenosis

than half of the functioning nephrons. Thus, in unilateral RAS, an abnormal serum creatinine level suggests concomitant dysfunction of the contralateral "nonstenosed" kidney, and angioplasty most probably will not contribute to improvement or preservation of renal function *(Table 3)*.

However, a recent study suggested, that renal angioplasty can be offered to a broader group of patients, even with elevated creatinine levels in unilateral RAS. Ongoing randomized trials hopefully will provide further evidence.

Angiography remains the "gold standard" for the evaluation of RAS. Using 4-F equipment and 20 ml of contrast media or even gadolinium for a diagnostic angiography in digital subtraction technique, this examination has a negligible complication rate. First step of the examination is to obtain a semi-selective overview with the use of a short pigtail catheter. Thus, potential accessory renal arteries, which have an incidence of about 25%, will be visualized. Due to the origin of the right renal artery slightly more ventrally and the left renal artery more dorsally, the ostia of both renal arteries are normally best visualized at a 20° LAO projection. After this step we proceed with a right coronary Judkins 4 or a Cobra catheter for selective angiography. In severely caudally angulated arteries it is sometimes helpful to use a recurved catheter like a Shepherd's Hook, a Sidewinder-1 (different vendors) or an SOS Omni Selective catheter (AngioDynamics, Glens Falls, NY, USA). Whether an angiographic stenosis of 50% or ≥ 70% should be considered a significant lesion is a matter of ongoing debate.

> **TIPS AND TRICKS**
>
> ▪ *Since the complication rate is negligible, there is no argument to be restrictive with the use of diagnostic angiography.*

Techniques for Renal Artery Angioplasty

Preinterventional measurement of the pressure gradient can be useful if angiography reveals a borderline stenosis. But measurement using a 4-F or 5-F diagnostic catheter should be avoided, first because of the hazard of plaque mobilization and embolization into the kidney, and second because the pressure gradient might show falsely elevated results in tighter stenosis using a diagnostic catheter leading to an obstruction of the artery.

New miniaturized pressure wires showed a correlation of a mean pressure gradient of 20 mmHg with an angiographic stenosis of 50%. This could be an argument for the significance of these stenoses. Other authors even consider a mean pressure gradient of 15 or even 10 mmHg to be indicative of a hemodynamic relevance.

Several techniques were developed for renal interventions, some have the character of a peripheral intervention using stiff 0.035" guide wires, others resemble coronary interventions operating with 0.014" wires and low-profile equipment.

Guide Wire Technique

This technique needs two puncture sites, one for the guiding catheter, and one for a pigtail or different catheter to prove the correct position of the balloon and stent. Using this technique, a stiff 0.018" or 0.035" guide wire is introduced in the renal artery over a 5-F diagnostic catheter. Then, the catheter is exchanged for a balloon catheter for predilatation and, finally, the stent is inserted *(Figure 1)*. Each step can be checked by angiography via the pigtail catheter. Disadvantage of this technique is the need for two puncture sites.

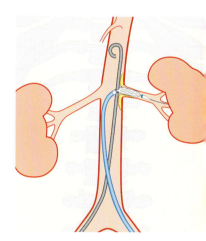

FIGURE 1.
Guide wire technique. Stent implantation, position confirmed via the pigtail catheter.

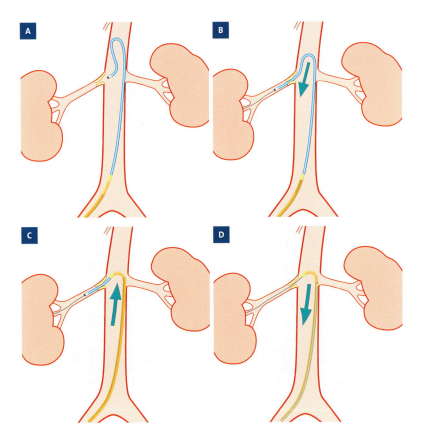

FIGURES 2A TO 2D.
a) Cannulation of the renal artery using a 5-F Sidewinder or SOS Omni Selective diagnostic catheter via a 6-F or 7-F guiding catheter.
b) After passage of the stenosis with a stiff guide wire (0.018" or 0.035"), the diagnostic catheter is pulled into the artery (eventually after predilatation).
c) Now the guiding catheter can easily be advanced over the diagnostic catheter to the ostium of the renal artery.
d) The diagnostic catheter is removed.

> **TIPS AND TRICKS**
>
> ▪ Passage of the stenosis with a catheter or sheath before stenting should be avoided because of the risk of plaque embolization.

Coaxial Technique

This technique can be successfully used in severely angled renal arteries via a femoral approach. A 5-F Sidewinder-1 catheter or a 5-F SOS Omni Selective catheter™ (AngioDynamics® Inc., Glens Falls, NY, USA) is advanced through a 7-F guiding catheter. After passage of the RAS with a stiff 0.035" or 0.018" guide wire, the diagnostic catheter is first introduced through the stenosis followed by the guiding catheter. Recurved diagnostic catheters provide a mechanical advantage for this maneuver, since they are pulled down the aorta for passage of the stenosis, thereby exerting greater axial force across the lesion. After the guiding catheter is in place, the diagnostic catheter can be withdrawn and the angioplasty carried out *(Figure 2)*. This technique, in our opinion, harbors the risk of severe atheroembolism and should be avoided, since highly angulated renal arteries can easily be recanalized via a brachial or even radial approach.

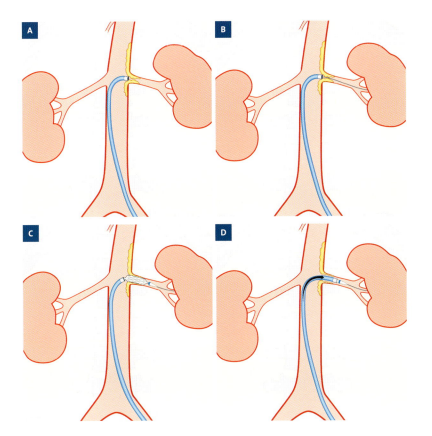

FIGURES 3A TO 3D.
a) Positioning of an RDC (or IMA) guiding catheter at the ostium of the renal artery.
b) Passage of the stenosis with a 0.014" guide wire.
c) Direct stent implantation (predilatation optional). Enough space should be left between the stent and the tip of the guiding catheter to avoid distal displacement of the stent during inflation.
d) For safe retrieval of the balloon, the guiding catheter can be advanced into the stent.

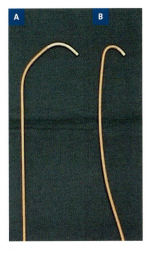

FIGURES 4A AND 4B.
a) RDC (renal double curve) guiding catheter.
b) IMA (internal mammary artery) guiding catheter.

Guiding-Catheter Technique

This is, in our opinion, the technique of first choice, since stents and balloons with improved flexibility and lower profile are available *(Figure 3)*. With a femoral approach we recommend the use of a 7-F RDC (renal double curve) catheter (Guidant, Cordis, Boston Scientific). In more angulated arteries or in case of an abdominal aorta with a small diameter a 7-F IMA (internal mammary artery) catheter can be of advantage *(Figure 4)*. In severely angulated arteries *(Figure 5)* or in case of high-grade obstructive disease or severe kinking of the pelvic or lower abdominal artery a 7-F multipurpose catheter via the brachial approach is recommended *(Figure 6)*. Using the new rapid-exchange stent systems, a 0.014" floppy-tipped coronary guide wire (e.g., Galeo ES™,

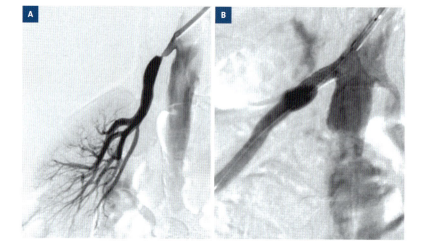

FIGURES 5A AND 5B.
a) Subtotal stenosis in a severely angulated artery.
b) Stenting via a brachial approach.

FIGURES 6A TO 6C.
a) High-grade stenosis of left renal artery in a severely diseased lower abdominal aorta.
b, c) Recanalization via a brachial approach.

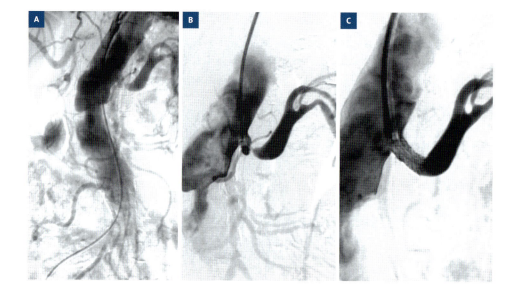

Biotronik, Berlin, Germany) can be chosen, which allows for easy passage of even very tight stenoses with a minimized risk of subintimal wire placement.

In our experience, with this technique the lowest intervention and radiation time can be achieved.

Balloon Angioplasty and Stenting

Several registries and one randomized trial have shown, that stent implantation in ostial stenoses is mandatory for achieving a high primary success rate and low restenosis rate. Ostial stenoses tend to be severely calcified, and often show significant recoil after balloon angioplasty. Late restenosis potentially occurs partly by progression of atherosclerotic plaque of the aorta into the ostium of the renal artery. Therefore in proximal and ostial stenoses stent deployment should be carried out with 1–2 mm of the stent extending into the opacified aortic lumen to prevent plaque protrusion into the renal artery.

In truncal stenosis or stenosis involving side branches, balloon angioplasty can be sufficient and stenting is reserved for unsatisfactory primary results. In bifurcational stenoses a kissing wire technique is recommended to protect against inadvertent plaque shifting, which can lead to an occlusion of one of the involved arteries. Since kissing stent implantation might be carried out, an 8-F guiding catheter is necessary *(Figure 7)*. Alternatively, two separate arterial access sites can be chosen.

In fibromuscular dysplasia balloon angioplasty alone yields sufficient short- and long-term results in almost all cases. Balloons should not be oversized with the goal to achieve an angiographically optimal result, since the typical "string of beads" appearance is often unchanged after angioplasty, although the stenoses are eliminated *(Figure 8)*.

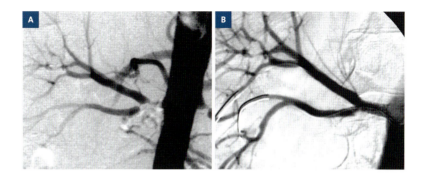

FIGURES 7A TO 7D.

a) High-grade bifurcational or side-branch stenosis.
b) Unsatisfactory result after balloon angioplasty of the side branch.
c) Kissing stent technique.
d) Optimal result.

TIPS AND TRICKS

- Low-profile equipment should be preferred for RAS angioplasty.

Figures 8a and 8b.

Typical appearance of fibromuscular dysplasia a) before and b) after balloon angioplasty.

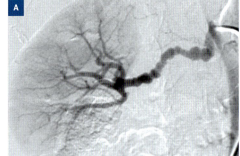 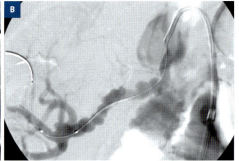

Figure 9.

Long subtotal renal stenosis requiring predilatation.

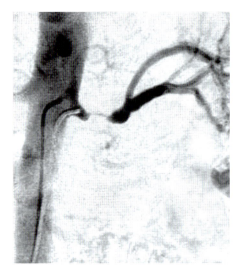

The introduction of new low-profile stents changed the character of renovascular intervention. Former balloon-expandable stents were replaced, which required stiffer 0.018" or 0.035" guide wires and predilatation or protected deployment after passage of the stenosis with the guiding catheter because of low flexibility and unsatisfactory passing profile. Several low-profile, rapid-exchange, balloon-premounted stents for renal artery stenting are now available. The RX Herculink plus™ stent (Guidant-ACS Inc. Temecula, CA, USA) was the first of these stents on the market. It is a 0.014" guide wire-compatible system available in stent diameters of 4.0–7.0 mm in 0.5-mm intervals and stent lengths of 12 mm and 18 mm. It

TABLE 4.

	Stent diameter (mm)	Stent length (mm)	Working length (cm)	Maximal guide wire (inch)	Vendor
Herculink™	4.0–7.0	12, 18	80, 135	0.014	Guidant
Hippocampus™	4.0–7.0	10, 15, 20, 24	80, 145	0.014	Invatec
Palmaz Genesis™ on Amiia™	4.0–7.0	12, 15, 18, 24	80, 142	0.014	Cordis
Express™ SD	4.0–7.0	15, 19	90, 150	0.018	Boston Scientific
Tsunami™ RX Peripheral stent	5.0–7.0	12/18	90, 150	0.018	Terumo
Racer	4.0–7.0	12, 18	80, 130	0.018	Medtronic
Radix	5.0–7.0	12, 17	75, 135	0.018	Sorin

TABLE 4. *Low-profile stents for renal artery angioplasty.*

was followed by several other devices *(Table 4)*. For most of these stents a 6-F guiding catheter is required, but a 7-F guiding catheter is recommended for better visualization of the stent position during deployment.

With low-profile stents even in subtotal stenoses predilatation is not necessary with the exception of longer subtotal stenoses *(Figure 9)*. Since the balloons are often slightly longer than the stent, dissection of the renal artery at the distal end of the stent can occur. This complication can be avoided if the implantation is started with a low pressure (6–8 atm) and finished with higher pressure (10–14 atm) after retrieval of the balloon for some millimeters into the stent.

Some interventionalists recommend measurement of the vessel diameter or predilatation for determination of the exact vessel size. The presence of a poststenotic dilatation, which is frequent in RAS, can complicate the choice of the exact stent size, especially in ostial stenoses *(Figure 10)*.

> **TIPS AND TRICKS**
>
> ■ *Normal renal artery diameter is 6.0–6.5 mm for men and 5.5–6.0 mm for women.*

Summary

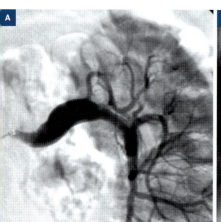 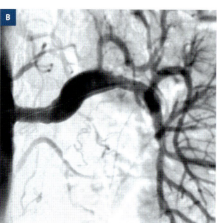

FIGURES 10A AND 10B.
a) High-grade stenosis with severe poststenotic dilatation.
b) Result after implantation of a 6.5/18-mm stent.

If postdilatation is necessary, a Submarine Rapido™ (Invatec, Roncadelle, Italy) or an Ultra-soft™ SV (Boston Scientific Corp., Natick, MA, USA) is suitable. Overdilatation can result in type B dissection or vessel rupture with fatal bleeding. During the dilatation process we always interview the patient for back pain. In case of vessel rupture the balloon should be reinserted and inflated with low pressure for several minutes. With this technique the rupture can seal and surgery will be avoided.

RAS is common and increasingly diagnosed. After the first enthusiastic acceptance of renal artery angioplasty, skepticism came up after randomized trials found no benefit concerning arterial hypertension after interventional therapy. But clinical experience and the fact, that these randomized trials showed several limitations, provide enough arguments to regard revascularization of RAS still as an effective therapy for many patients.

With special equipment RAS revascularization is very successful and shows a very low complication rate. Until more powerful randomized trials, especially focusing on renal dysfunction, will be published, renal angioplasty should further be offered to well-selected patients in many different clinical situations.

References

1. Beutler JJ, Van Ampting JMA, Van de Ven PJG, Koomans HA, Beek FJA, Woittiez AJJ, Mali WPTM. Long-term effects of arterial stenting on kidney function for patients with ostial atherosclerotic renal artery stenosis and renal insufficiency. J Am Soc Nephrol 2001;12:1475–81.
2. Blum U, Krumme B, Flugel P, et al. Treatment of ostial renal-artery stenoses with vascular endoprostheses after unsuccessful balloon angioplasty. N Engl J Med 1997;336:459–65.
3. Conlon PJ, O'Riordan E, Kalra PA. New insights into the epidemiologic and clinical manifestations of atherosclerotic renovascular disease. Am J Kidney Dis 2000;35:573–87.
4. Dorros G, Jaff M, Mathiak L, He T. Multicenter Palmaz stent renal artery stenosis revascularization registry report: four-year follow-up of 1,058 successful patients. Cathet Cardiovasc Interv 2002;55:182–8.
5. Harden PN, MacLeod MJ, Rodger RSC, Baxter GM, Connell JM, Dominiczak AF, et al. Effect of renal artery stenting on progression of renovascular failure. Lancet 1997;349:1133–6.
6. Rundback JH, Crea G, Rozenblit GN, Poplausky M, Maddineni S, Olson C. The difficult renal angioplasty. Cathet Cardiovasc Interv 2001;52:120–6.
7. Safian RD, Textor SC. Renal-artery stenosis. N Engl J Med 2001;344:431–42.
8. Van de Ven PJG, Kaatee R, Beutler JJ, Beek FJA, Woittiez AJJ, Buskens E, Koomans HA, Mali WPT. Arterial stenting and balloon angioplasty in ostial atherosclerotic renovascular disease: a randomised trial. Lancet 1999;353:282–6.
9. Van Jaarsveld BC, Krijnen P, Pieterman H, Derkx FHM, Deinum J, Postma CT, Dees A, Woittiez AJJ, Bartelink AKM, Man In 'T Veld AJ, Schalekamp MADH. The effect of balloon angioplasty on hypertension in atherosclerotic renal-artery stenosis. N Engl J Med 2000;342:1007–14.
10. Watson PS, Hadjipetrou P, Cox SV, Piemonte TC, Eisenhauer AC. Effect of renal artery stenting on renal function and size in patients with atherosclerotic renovascular disease. Circulation 2000;102:1671–7.
11. Zeller T, Frank U, Muller C, Burgelin K, Sinn L, Bestehorn HP, Cook-Bruns N, Neumann FJ. Predictors of improved renal function after percutaneous stent-supported angioplasty of severe atherosclerotic ostial artery stenosis. Circulation 2003;108:2244–9.

Chapter Six

Endovascular Therapy of Aneurysms and Dissections of the Thoracic Aorta

A. Endovascular Therapy of Thoracic Aortic Aneurysms and Aortic Rupture

The topographic distribution of aortic aneurysms indicates that only 20% occur in the thoracic segment, whereas 80% are localized in the abdominal part of the aorta. Data on the natural history of throracic aortic aneurysms show a survival rate of 65% after 1 year and 20% after 5 years without surgical therapy, stressing the clinical relevance of this disease.

Surgical repair of thoracic aortic aneurysms is particularly challenging in lesions of the descending thoracic aorta. In general, mortality rates are depending on the etiology and the extent of the lesion as well as on coexistent morbidity. Elective repair of thoracic aortic aneurysms shows mortality rates ranging between 5–15%. In case of emergency procedures for ruptured aneurysms or dissections, mortality rates may exceed 50%.

Endovascular stent-graft placement has been proposed as a treatment alternative for aneurysms and dissections involving the descending thoracic aorta. Although data from large randomized trials are pending, the technique is generally considered to be an effective and less invasive treatment option in case of suitable morphologic conditions, particularly in high-risk patients with significant comorbidity.

Clinical Manifestation and Noninvasive Workup

Patients with chronic descending thoracic aortic aneurysms are usually asymptomatic. The diagnosis is made incidentally during routine chest X-ray or computed tomography (CT; *Figure 1*). Large aneurysms may provoke symptoms related to compression of surrounding structures, e.g., difficult swallowing related to compression of the esophagus or breathing abnormalities as well as recurrent bronchopulmonary infections due to bronchus compression. Thoracic pain is rare in uncomplicated aneurysms, it typically occurs in patients with pending or acute rupture or dissection. In these patients, hemodynamic depression with signs of hemorrhagic shock is a typical condition which requires immediate therapy. However, a relevant percentage of

CONTENTS DVD

12. Endovascular repair of a descending thoracic aortic aneurysm (06:37 min)
13. Stent-graft implantation for type B aortic dissection (11:22 min)

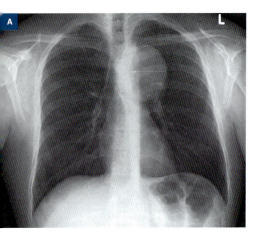 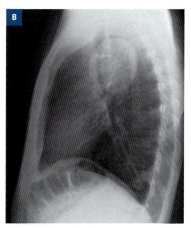 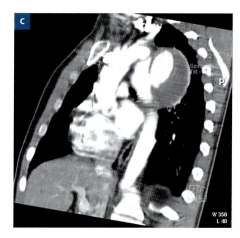

Figures 1a to 1c.

a) Chest X-ray of a 31-year-old male patient 9 months after a motorcycle accident, posterior-anterior view.
b) Lateral view.
c) CT reconstruction showing a partially thrombosed post-traumatic false aneurysm "in loco typico".

patients may present with hypertensive conditions requiring intensive antihypertensive therapy, preferably using i.v. β-blockers.

In our practice, the definitive diagnosis is mainly based on contrast-enhanced spiral CT. Besides characterization of the lesion by maximum aneurysm diameter and length, diameters of the proximal and distal reference aortic segment are obtained for sizing of the endoprosthesis.

Additional information obtained by the CT scan includes the presence of thrombotic material and calcium in the aneurysmal sac and in the reference aortic segments. In general, descending thoracic aortic aneurysms can be considered appropriate for endovascular repair, if there is a sufficient proximal neck of at least 15 mm to the origin of the left subclavian artery. Further limitations are related to the diameters of the commercially available endoprostheses, which range from 24 to 46 mm. Considering a recommended oversizing of the endoprosthesis by 2–4 mm, reference aortic diameters between 20 and 44 mm are treatable.

An important precondition for endovascular repair is a diameter of the iliac vessels of at least 7 mm, allowing the insertion of the delivery device (22–27 F). Therefore, in all patients the anatomic status of the access vessels has to be investigated prior to the implantation procedure by intraarterial digital subtraction angiography (DSA).

Endovascular Procedure

In our institute, all stent-graft procedures are carried out in the angiography suite under general anesthesia (Figures 2a and 2b).

Using a left brachial approach, a 5-F angiographic pigtail catheter is initially advanced into the ascending aorta. This catheter allows contrast injection during the procedure and helps to identify the origin of the left subclavian artery, which is an important anatomic landmark for positioning of the stent graft *(Figure 3c)*.

Routinely, mechanical injections of 25 ml nonionic contrast media with a flow rate of 15 ml/s are used.

Furthermore, the common femoral artery is surgically exposed. In case of insufficient diameter of the access vessels or severe calcification, surgical exposure of the common iliac artery may be necessary before cannulation.

After achieving vascular access, 5,000 units of heparin sodium are administered intravenously. A 5-F diagnostic multipurpose catheter is first advanced over a soft wire into the ascending aorta. The wire is then exchanged for an ultrastiff guide wire (Meyer Extra Back-up 0.035" x 300 cm or Lunderquist, Cook, 0.035" x 300 cm) to facilitate the introduction and delivery of the stent graft.

The endoprosthesis commonly used is the Valiant device (former Talent; Medtronic, World Medical Manufacturing Corp, Sunrise, FL, USA). This self-expanding endoprosthesis consists of circumferential nitinol stent springs arranged as a tube for conformance to the lumen and covered on its exterior with a Dacron graft. For implantation, the Valiant endoprosthesis is compressed in a polytetrafluoroethylene (PTFE) sheath with an outer diameter of 22–27 F. For deployment, the endoprosthesis is fixed in position with a pusher, while the sheath is withdrawn.

To achieve an optimal positioning of the endoprosthesis, it is advisable to start deployment of the proximal bare springs and of the first covered ring in the aortic arch after controlling the position by contrast injection *(Figure 3c)*.

After pullback of the endoprosthesis to the desired location, the rest of the endoprosthesis can be released *(Figure 3d)*. In all cases, postdilatations with a compliant aortic balloon catheter (Reliant, Medtronic) are performed in the covered part of the endoprostheses to achieve an optimal alignment of the graft material to the aortic wall.

Postinterventional Treatment and Follow-Up

After surgical closure of the access site, no additional anticoagulation is required. Routinely, 100 mg ASA/day is given to the patients. All patients are enrolled in a follow-up protocol including clinical examinations and CT scans before hospital discharge, at 3 and 12 months, and yearly thereafter *(Figure 3e)*.

FIGURES 2A AND 2B.
Endovascular stent-graft placement for treatment of descending thoracic aortic aneurysms.

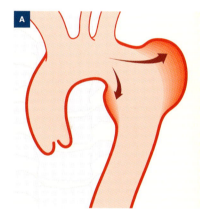

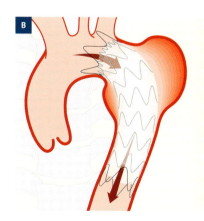

Specific Cases

FIGURES 3A TO 3E.
a) Aneurysm of the descending thoracic aorta – angiography.
b) CT reconstruction.
c) positioning of the Talent endoprosthesis.
d) angiographic result after implantation of the endoprosthesis.
e) CT reconstruction at 3-months follow-up.

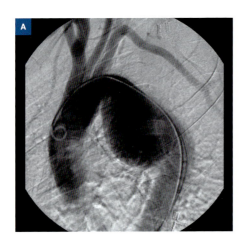

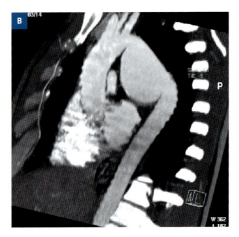

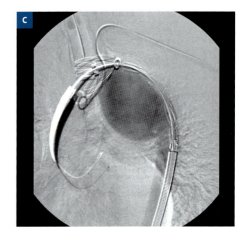

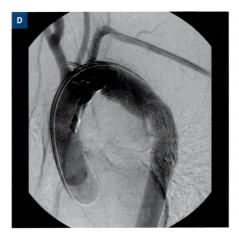

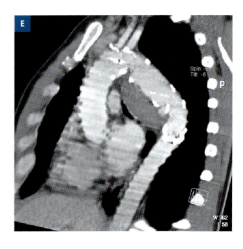

Summary of Outcome Results

Stent-Graft Treatment for Descending Thoracic Aortic Aneurysms

In 1999, Mitchell et al. published a single-center experience in 103 patients (mean age 69 years) undergoing first-generation stent-graft repair of descending thoracic aortic aneurysms. The stent graft was home made using self-expanding "Z"-stents covered by a woven Dacron tube graft.

Complete aneurysm thrombosis was achieved in 86 patients (83%). Early mortality, defined as a death during the same hospitalization or in <30 days, was $9 \pm 3\%$, and was associated with relevant perioperative cerebrovascular accident (CVA) or myocardial infarction. Major perioperative morbidity occurred in 31 patients, and included paraplegia in three, CVA in seven, and respiratory insufficiency in twelve cases. Actuarial survival was $81 \pm 4\%$ at 1 year, and $73 \pm 5\%$ at 2 years. Treatment failure (including all late, sudden, unexplained deaths) occurred in 38 patients, and only $53 \pm 10\%$ of patients were free of complication at 3.7 years. Five patients required late operative therapy for endoleaks associated with aneurysm enlargement.

Meanwhile, stent-graft technology has substantially improved. Currently, standardized devices with various diameters and lengths are available allowing immediate treatment of up to 80% of the lesions in the descending thoracic aorta.

Between 1999 and March 2003, 47 patients (31 male, mean age 67.3 years) underwent elective endovascular repair of descending thoracic aortic aneurysms in our institution. In total, 67 endoprostheses (Talent, Medtronic, n = 57; Excluder, Gore, n = 10) were implanted (eleven patients with two, seven patients with three, two patients with four endoprostheses).

Endoprosthesis implantation was successfully performed in all cases without periinterventional complications. In eight of the 47 patients, a partial residual perfusion of the aneurysmal sac could be demonstrated during the postinterventional CT. However, in only two patients a relevant type 1 endoleak was detected, which could be treated successfully by implantation of a second endoprosthesis. In the remaining patients, the CT control at 1 month revealed that in all cases the aneurysmal sac was completely thrombosed without further treatment. There were no procedure-associated deaths. Postinterventionally, transient renal failure occurred in five patients (10.6%). In one patient, clinical signs of a minor stroke with transient weakness in the right arm were observed. The cerebral CT at 3 days showed no detectable ischemic lesion. The symptoms resolved completely after 12 h. There were no cases of paraplegia or death and no instances of rupture or leakages during the subsequent average follow-up period of 14 months.

These results suggest that with currently available stent grafts, aneurysmatic lesions of the descending thoracic aorta can be treated effectively. Midterm results are promising, but the potential of late endoleak development, as seen in other vessel areas, remains a concern.

Endovascular Repair of Acute Aortic Rupture

Perforating lesions of the descending thoracic aorta are a life-threatening clinical condition associated with high morbidity and mortality. Between January 1999 and October 2003, a total of 31 patients (19 male, mean age 62.1 years) underwent endovascular treatment for perforating lesions in the descending aorta at the Heart Center of the University of Leipzig.

In 21 cases (group A), the aortic perforation was due to ruptured aortic type B dissections (n = 7) or rupture of preexisting atherosclerotic thoracic aneurysms (n = 14) *(Figure 4a to 4d)*.

Ten patients (group B) were treated for posttraumatic perforations of the descending aorta. In total, 42 endoprostheses were implanted (seven patients with two, two patients with three endoprostheses).

The implantation of the endoprostheses was successfully performed in all cases without periinterventional complications. In one case, implantation of a second endoprosthesis became

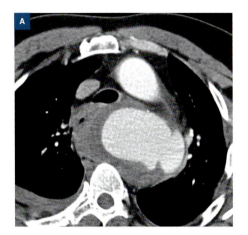 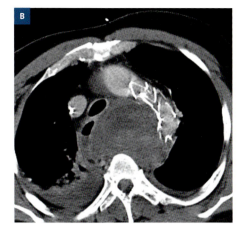

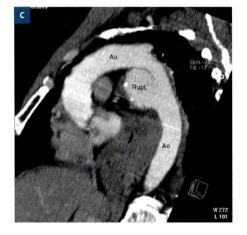

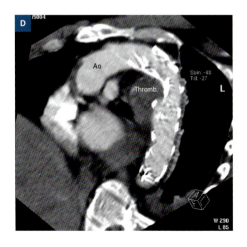

necessary due to incomplete coverage of the lesion with subsequent leakage. Three of the 31 patients died within 30 days (9.7%). All deaths occurred in group A, corresponding to a mortality rate of 14.3% in this group versus 0% in group B. Similarly, postinterventional complications were more prevalent in group A with 28.6% (renal failure n = 4; ischemic stroke n = 2) versus 10.0% in group B (renal failure n = 1). In both groups, there were no cases of paraplegia or further death and no instances of rupture during the average follow-up period of 17 months.

According to these data, interventional stent-graft repair offers an effective treatment option for emergency treatment of descending aortic perforations. The procedure-associated morbidity and mortality are higher for patients with ruptured dissecting or atherosclerotic thoracic aneurysms than for traumatic aortic disruptions.

FIGURES 4A TO 4D.

a) Acute rupture of a chronic descending thoracic aortic aneurysm with contrast extravasation into the mediastinum (Rupt) and relevant hemorrhagic mediastinal and pleural effusion.
b) Complete thrombosis of the mediastinal hematoma after sealing of the perforation by implantation of a stent-graft prosthesis.
c) Two-dimensional CT reconstruction (multiplanar reconstruction) before and
d) after successful stent-graft repair (LAO-like view).

B. Endovascular Therapy of Type B Aortic Dissections

Acute aortic dissection is one of the most serious and dramatic pathologies. The incidence is estimated at ten to 20 cases per million population per year. If the condition is left untreated, the mortality is 36–72% within 48 h of diagnosis, and 62–91% die within 1 week after the onset of symptoms.

Figure 5 shows commonly used classifications of aortic dissection based on the involvement of the ascending and descending aorta. Because of its prognostic significance, the Stanford classification is most commonly used. As acute type A aortic dissection is associated with a mortality rate of 1–2% per hour during the first 24 h and about 80% during the first 2 weeks, immediate surgical repair with replacement of the ascending aorta and, if necessary, of the aortic valce and the aortic arch is mandatory.

While around 60% of all dissections are classified as type A according to the Stanford classification, about 40% of dissections involve exclusively the descending thoracic aorta, and are therefore classified as type B dissections. Due to the unsatisfactory results of surgical reconstruction with mortality rates up to 50% after 1 year, medical therapy including the use of β-blockers and other antihypertensive drugs is the preferred treatment. Nevertheless, the mortality rate among patients who receive medical therapy for type B dissection remains about 20%. The persistence of pulsatile blood flow through the proximal entry into the false channel pedisposes the patient to a sequence of dangerous events such as aortic aneurysm formation, organ or peripheral ischemia caused by obstruction of primary aortic branch vessels or the true lumen and, finally, aortic rupture.

After the positive experience with grafting TAA, this technique was extended to type B aortic dissection. The

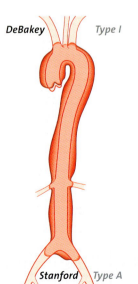

FIGURE 5. *For aortic dissection two classification systems predominate – the DeBakey and the Stanford classification. In both systems, aortic dissections with and without ascending aortic involvement are distinguished for prognostic and therapeutic reasons.*

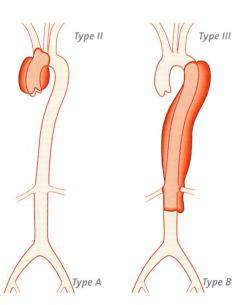

rationale for this endovascular technique is the endovascular sealing of the proximal entry sites by implantation of a stent-graft endoprosthesis *(Figure 6)*, thereby inducing thrombosis of the false channel. As a result of sealing the proximal entry site, the false channel is likely to collapse and thrombose, a process that mimics the natural healing process and may eventually lead to reconstruction and remodeling of the entire aorta *(see Figure 7)*.

Clinical Manifestation and Noninvasive Workup

In contrast to patients with descending thoracic aortic aneurysms which are usually asymptomatic, patients with type B aortic dissections present with sudden onset of severe thoracic pain, which may radiate into the spine area. In many cases, this event may be related to an episode of severe hypertension. As most patients have a typical cardiovascular risk profile, differentiation from acute coronary syndroms may be difficult. In some cases with extensive dissection, additional symptoms including signs of peripheral or visceral ischemia or renal failure may be related to the compression of the true lumen or important abdominal side branches of the aorta.

In general, diagnosis and classification of aortic dissection are mainly based on contrast-enhanced spiral CT. Besides the localization of the proximal entry tear, important information about the size of the false and true lumen, the involvement of the abdominal aorta and pelvic arteries, and the perfusion state of the renal and visceral arteries can be obtained.

Additional diagnostic tools include transesophageal echocardiography which may be helpful for the detection of entry tears and can be used throughout the interventional procedure for guidance of stent-graft delivery. Furthermore, intraarterial DSA is very helpful to assess the origin of abdominal aortic side branches as well as the status of the access vessels.

In general, type B aortic dissections can be considered appropriate for endovascular repair, if the dissection does not involve parts of the aortic arch and if there is an identifiable proximal entry tear. With regard to the involvement of the aortic side branches, origin of one renal artery from the false channel is a frequent finding which is not considered a contraindication for endovascular treatment. In case of involvement of both renal arteries or of relevant visceral side branches, the indication should be discussed carefully on a case-by-case basis.

> **TIPS AND TRICKS**
>
> ▪ *To avoid distal redissection, do not oversize the endoprosthesis by more than 2 mm and avoid postdilatation of the distal end.*

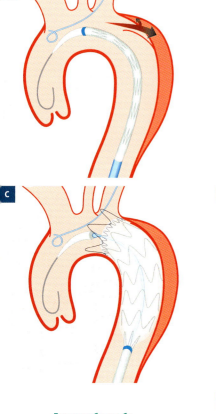
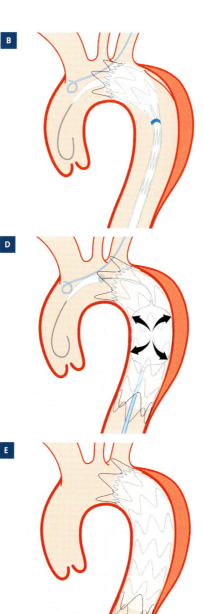

Figures 6a to 6e.
Endovascular stent-graft placement for treatment of type B aortic dissections.
a) Introduction of the stent-graft device.
b) Release of the proximal two segments and pullback of the device into the desired location.
c) Full release of the device.
d) Optional postdilatation only in the proximal part of the prosthesis.
e) Final result.

Endovascular Procedure

In general, the endovascular stent-graft procedure, which is outlined in Figure 6, follows the same steps as described for the treatment of thoracic aneurysms.

Again it is important to mention, that for optimal positioning of the endoprosthesis it is advisable to start deployment of the proximal bare springs and the first covered ring in the aortic arch followed by pullback of the endoprosthesis to the desired location *(Figure 6b)*. A full coverage of the proximal entry tear must be achieved which can be checked during the procedure by continuous transesophageal echocardiography monitoring. Postdilatations should only be performed in case of incomplete alignment of the endoprosthesis in the proximal part. Postdilatations in the distal part of the endoprosthesis are not recommended due to the risk of creating a new entry tear.

Postinterventional treatment follows the same guidelines as described for thoracic aortic aneurysms.

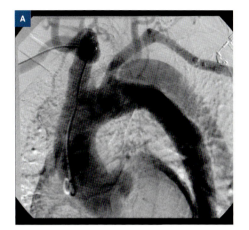
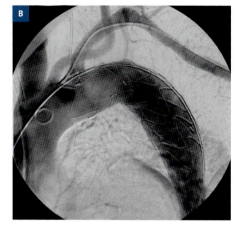
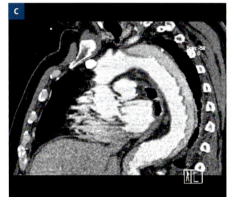
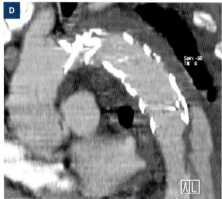
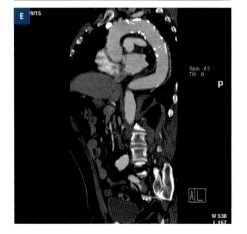

Specific Cases

FIGURES 7A TO 7E.
a) Type B aortic dissection.
b) Complete sealing after stent-graft implantation.
c) CT reconstructions preinterventional.
d) CT reconstruction 2 days after stent-graft implantation showing thrombosis of the proximal false channel.
e) CT reconstruction at 1-year follow-up showing complete remodeling of the aortic wall.

Summary of Outcome Results

In 1999, Nienaber et al. published the first systematic investigation of endovascular stent-graft treatment for acute type B aortic dissections. They prospectively evaluated the safety and efficacy of elective transluminal endovascular stent-graft insertion in twelve consecutive patients with descending (type B) aortic dissection and compared the results with surgery in twelve matched controls. In all 24 patients, aortic dissection was diagnosed by magnetic resonance angiography. In each group, the dissection involved the aortic arch in three patients and the descending thoracic aorta in all twelve patients. With the patient under general anesthesia, either surgical resection was undertaken or a custom-designed endovascular stent graft was placed by unilateral arteriotomy.

Stent-graft placement resulted in no morbidity or mortality, whereas surgery for type B dissection was associated with four deaths (33%; p = 0.09) and five serious adverse events (42%; p = 0.04) within 12 months. Transluminal placement of the stent-graft prosthesis was successful in all patients, and no leakage occurred. Sealing of the entry tear was monitored during the procedure by transesophageal ultrasonography and angiography, and thrombosis of the false lumen was confirmed by magnetic resonance imaging in all twelve patients after a mean of 3 months. There were no deaths or paraplegia, stroke, embolization, side-branch occlusion, or infection in the stent-graft group. All patients who received stent grafts, and seven patients who underwent surgery for type B dissection (58%; p = 0.04) recovered completely.

A recently published meta-analysis by Eggebrecht et. al. evaluated data from 39 studies involving 609 patients with regard to the clinical success, complications, and outcomes of endovascular stent-graft placement for patients with descending aortic dissection. Procedural success was reported in 98.2% of patients. Major complications were reported in 11.1%. Periprocedural stroke was encountered more frequently than paraplegia (1.9% vs. 0.8%). Overall complications were significantly higher in patients undergoing stent-graft placement for acute aortic dissection than in patients with chronic aortic dissection (21.7% ± 2.8% vs. 9.1% ± 2.3%; P = 0.005). The overall 30-day mortality was 5.3%, and was three-fold higher in patients with acute aortic dissection when compared with chronic aortic dissection (9.8% vs. 3.2%, P = 0.015). In addition, 2.8% of patients died over a mean follow-up period of 19.5 ± 7.1 months. Kaplan-Meier analysis yielded overall survival rates of 90.6% at 6 months, 89.9% at 1 year, and 88.8% at 2 years, respectively.

These preliminary observations suggest that elective, nonsurgical insertion of an endovascular stent graft is safe and effective in selected patients showing thoracic aortic dissection. The overall prognostic advantage of stent-graft treatment over medical therapy for uncomplicated type B aortic dissection is currently under investigation in the INSTEAD trial.

References

1. Alric P, Berthet JP, Branchereau P, Veerapen R, Marty-Ane CH. Endovascular repair for acute rupture of the descending thoracic aorta. J Endovasc Ther 2002; 9:II-51–9.
2. Attar S, Cardarelli MG, Downing SW, Rodriguez A, Wallace DC, West RS, McLaughlin JS. Traumatic aortic rupture: recent outcome with regard to neurologic deficit. Ann Thorac Surg 1999;67:959–65.
3. Cambria RP, Brewster DC, Gertler J, Moncure AC, Gusberg R, Tilson MD, Darling RC, Hammond G, Mergeman J, Abbo. Vascular complications associated with spontaneous aortic dissection. J Vasc Surg 1988; 7:199–209.
4. Dake MD, Kato N, Mitchell RS, Semba CP, Razavi MK, Shimono T, Hirano T, Takeda K, Yada I, Miller DC. Endovascular stent-graft placement for the treatment of acute aortic dissection. N Engl J Med 1999;340: 1546–52.
5. Eggebrecht H, Nienaber CA, Neuhauser M, Baumgart D, Kische S, Schmermund A, Herold U, Rehders TC, Jakob HG, Erbel R. Endovascular stent-graft placement in aortic dissection: a meta-analysis. Eur Heart J. 2006;27:489–98.
6. Erbel R, Alfonso F, Boileau C, Dirsch O, Eber B, Haverich A, Rakowski H, Struyven J, Radegran K, Sechtem U, Taylor J, Zollikofer C, Klein WW, Mulder B, Providencia LA. Diagnosis and management of aortic dissection. Recommendations of the Task Force on Aortic Dissection, European Society of Cardiology. Eur Heart J 2001;22:1642–81.
7. Gorich J, Asquan Y, Seifarth H, Kramer S, Kapfer X, Orend KH, Sunder-Plassmann L, Pamler R. Initial experience with intentional stent-graft coverage of the subclavian artery during endovascular thoracic aortic repairs. J Endovasc Ther 2002;9:II-39–43.
8. Hagan PG, Nienaber CA, Isselbacher EM, Bruckman D, Karavite DJ, Russman PL, Evangelista A, Fattori R, Suzuki T, Oh JK, Moore AG, Malouf JF, Pape LA, Gaca C, Sechtem U, Lenferik S, Deutsch HJ, Diedrichs H, Marcos y Rohles J, Llovet A, Gilon D, Das SK, Armstrong WF, Deeb GM, Eagle KA. The International Registry of acute Aortic Dissection (IRAD) – new insights into an old disease. JAMA 2000;283:897–903.
9. Johansson G, Markstrom U, Swedenborg J. Ruptured thoracic aortic aneurysms: a study of incidence and mortality rates. J Vasc Surg 1995;21:985–8.
10. Kato M, Matsuda T, Kaneko M, Kuratani T, Mizushima T, Seo Y, Uchida H, Kichikawa K, Maeda M, Ohnishi K. Outcomes of stent-graft treatment of false lumen in aortic dissection. Circulation 1998;19:II-305-12.
11. Koschyk DH, Meinertz T, Nienaber CA. Images in cardiovascular medicine. Intravascular ultrasound for stent implantation in aortic dissection. Circulation 2000;102:480–1.
12. Lemaire SA, Rice DC, Schmittling ZC, Coselli JS. Emergency surgery for thoracoabdominal aortic aneurysms with acute presentation. J Vasc Surg 2002;35:1171–8.
13. Lobato AC, Quick RC, Phillips B, Vranic M, Rodriguez-Lopez J, Douglas M, Diethrich EB. Immediate endovascular repair for descending thoracic aortic transsection secondary to blunt trauma. J Endovasc Ther 2000;7:16–20.
14. Miller DC, Mitchell RS, Oyer PE. Independent determinants of operative mortality for patients with aortic dissection. Circulation 1984;70:Suppl I:I-153–64.
15. Mitchell RS, Miller DC, Dake MD, Semba CP, Moore KA, Sakai T. Thoracic aortic aneurysm repair with an endovascular stent-graft: the "first generation". Ann Thorac Surg. 1999;67:1971–4.
16. Nienaber CA, Fattori R, Lund G, Dieckmann C, Wolf W, Kodolitsch Y von, Nicolas V, Piertangeli A. Nonsurgical reconstruction of thoracic aortic dissection by stent-graft placement. N Engl J Med 1999;340: 1539–45.
17. Oppel UO von, Dunne TT, DeGroot MK. Traumatic aortic rupture: twenty year metaanalysis of mortality and risk of paraplegia. Ann Thorac Surg 1994;58585–93.
18. Palambi M, Berardi F, Sposato S, Gargineo M, Bochicchio O, Iaria G, Leporelli P. Endovascular treatment of a ruptured thoracic aortic aneurysm. Eur J Vasc Endovasc Surg 2000;19:101–2.
19. Scheinert D, Krankenberg H, Schmidt A, Gummert JF, Nitzsche S, Scheinert S, Bräunlich S, Sorge I, Krakor R, Biamino G, Schuler G, Mohr FW. Endoluminal stent-graft placement for acute rupture of the descending thoracic aorta. Eur Heart J 2004;25: 694–700.
20. Schütz W, Gaus A, Meierhenrich R, Pamler R, Gorich J. Transesophageal echocardiographic guidance of thoracic aortic stent-graft implantation. J Endovasc Ther 2002;9:II-14–9.
21. Segesser LK von, Genoni M, Kunzli A. Surgery for ruptured thoracic thoraco-abdominal aortic aneurysms. Eur J Cardiothorac Surg 1996;10:996–1001.
22. Semba CP, Kato N, Kee ST, Lee GK, Mitchell RS, Miller DC, Dake MD. Acute rupture of the descending thoracic aorta: repair with use of endovascular stent-grafts. J Vasc Interv Radiol 1997;8:337–42.

Chapter Seven

*Endoluminal Treatment
of Abdominal
Aortic Aneurysm*

Introduction

Endovascular grafting represents a milestone in the treatment of patients with abdominal aortic aneurysm (AAA) in that it provided a treatment option for those patients deemed inoperable because of the presence of significant medical comorbidities.

Data from European Vascular & Endovascular Monitor (EVEM) in 2002 showed that endovascular procedures in Europe increased during the last 2 years and constitute about 10% of all aortic repairs. Clinical investigations confirmed that endovascular aneurysm repair (EVAR) is associated with decreased perioperative major morbidity, hospital stay, and recovery time compared to open surgery. Moreover, recent randomized clinical trials (DREAM, EVAR-1) demonstrated that an endovascular approach reduces perioperative mortality in patients at low risk compared to the results of standard surgery. However, it remains to be a concern, that the early benefit may be offset by a lower level of late clinical success that requires more intensive long-term surveillance, increased rates of reintervention, higher costs, and potential psychologic stress for the patients. Thus, in advocating endovascular treatment, especially in patients at low risk for operative repair, a critical analysis of late outcomes is required.

CONTENTS DVD

14. Endovascular repair of an abdominal aortic aneurysm (23:53 min)

Preinterventional Workup and Patient Selection

> **TIPS AND TRICKS**
>
> - During ultrasound examinations of patients with peripheral arterial disease, coronary artery disease or hypertension always screen for AAA.

Patients with AAA are usually asymptomatic, and diagnosis of the vascular lesion is made incidentally during abdominal ultrasound, angiography, or computed tomography (CT). In some cases with large aneurysms, a pulsating abdominal mass may be palpable. Abdominal pain radiating into the back is a rather rare finding in case of uncomplicated aneurysms and typically occurs in patients with impending or actual aneurysm rupture.

Patient selection is an important element in the complex equation of successful AAA endografting. Proper patient selection requires assessment of both physiologic and anatomic risk factors. The patient's age, cardiac, pulmonary, and renal function as well as the surgeon's experience and the hospital's volume all have an effect on the overall medical risk of elective surgical AAA repair. Specifically, data from large AAA repair series showed that patients >80 years had a 7.3% mortality rate after surgical aneurysm repair compared to 2.2% for patients <65 years. Therefore, open surgical repair is mainly considered for young, healthy patients, whereas endovascular stent grafting may be particularly beneficial for older and sicker patients who are otherwise no good candidates for surgical repair.

Based on a morphologic classification suggested by Allenberg et al., only aneurysms of category I, IIA and IIB are principally considered suitable for endovascular treatment *(Figure 1)*.

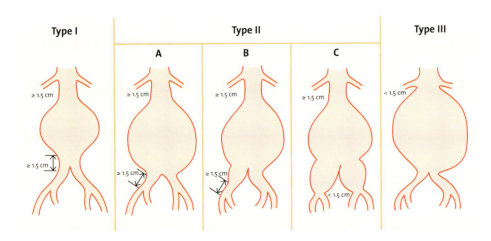

FIGURE 1.
Allenberg classification.

One major precondition is a sufficient proximal fixation zone. Generally, a cutoff value of 15 mm for the proximal aneurysm neck (distance between the renal arteries and the beginning of the aneurysm) is an accepted guideline. In fact, stable proximal fixation is the key to long-term AAA repair durability. The downward forces on the proximal attachment site are related to the diameter and curvature of the aorta. Increasing angulation of the proximal neck is associated with a significantly increased risk of type I endoleaks. As the degree of angulation increases, the proximal attachment area must lengthen. Patients with large or conical proximal aortic neck or with a layer of thrombus inside the neck are at higher risk of late failure.

A second major aspect is the morphologic situation of the distal landing zone in the iliac arteries. Heavily calcified iliac arteries can cause serious difficulties to the progression of the device. Therefore, a minimum access vessel diameter of at least 7 mm is required. The presence of a single aneurysm in a common iliac artery is not a contraindication provided that one hypogastric artery can be preserved. Distal deployment sites up to 20 mm in diameter can usually be utilized provided that reverse tapering of the iliac limb is achieved (bell-bottom technique). Deploying the device into the external iliac artery and occluding the ipsilateral hypogastric artery can exclude iliac vessels > 20 mm. However, this technique may be associated with risk of buttock, thigh, and pelvic claudication. In addition, a bilateral hypogastric occlusion should be avoided. Parlani et al. analyzed a series of 59 patients undergoing endovascular abdominal aneurysm repair with concomitant iliac aneurysm. In 33 patients, the internal iliac artery was also excluded to obtain aneurysm exclusion. After the procedure, five patients experienced buttock claudication (all occurring in patients with a covered or coiled internal iliac artery), whereas there were no cases of buttock or colon necrosis.

For assessment of the morphologic suitability and planning of the procedure, all patients are routinely examined with high-resolution contrast-enhanced spiral CT and intraarterial digital sub-

> **TIPS AND TRICKS**
>
> ▪ *In case of an angulated proximal neck the proximal attachment zone must be longer.*

traction angiography (DSA) using a calibrated 5-F pigtail catheter. *Figure 2* details typical measurements to describe the morphologic appearance and size of infrarenal aortic aneurysms. The following measurements are particularly important for selection of an appropriate endograft:

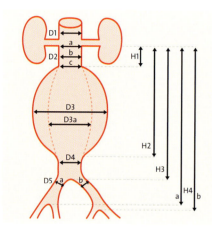

Figure 2.

D2 = diameter of the proximal fixation zone (proximal aneurysm neck);

D3 = maximum aneurysm diameter;

D5 = diameter of the distal fixation zone (separately measured for both iliac arteries);

H1 = length of proximal fixation zone (proximal aneurysm neck);

H3 = distance between the renal arteries and the aortic bifurcation;

H4 = distance between the renal arteries and the origin of the hypogastric arteries (separately measured for both iliac arteries) allowing calculation of the length of the common iliac arteries (H4 minus H3).

Available Stent-Graft Devices

Due to experience and improved graft technology, it is now possible to successfully treat aneurysms previously untreatable via endovascular approach. In the design of endoluminal devices for AAA repair, researchers have developed two different conceptual approaches.

The first type of stent grafts utilizes a miniaturized delivery system carrying a conventional, tubular, aortouniliac or bifurcated graft. An example of this type of device is the Ancure endograft (formerly EVT, Guidant, Menlo Park, CA, USA) made of Dacron with hooks at the extremities to ensure fixation, or the Endologix graft (Endologix, Irvine, CA, USA) made of polytetrafluoroethylene (PTFE) and fully stented.

The other type is a modular graft that is assembled inside the patient's body. Generally, modular grafts are fully stented, and the friction and radial force of the stent assure junction between segments. The stent is made of stainless steel, nitinol, an alloy of nickel and titanium, or elgiloy. In modular endografts, aortic fixation is achieved through the radial force of the covered stent over the infrarenal aortic neck with or without barbs, as in the AneuRx device (Medtronic, Santa Rosa, CA, USA), the Lifepath graft (Edwards, Irvine, CA, USA), and the Excluder graft (WL Gore and Associates, Flagstaff, AZ, USA). The Talent (Medtronic, Minneapolis, MN, USA), the Zenith (William Cook Europe, Bjaeverskov, Denmark), the Endofit (Endomed, Phoenix, AZ, USA), and the Quantum (Cordis, J & J, Warren, NJ, USA) devices have a bare stent (with or without hooks) over the top of the endograft that allows suprarenal fixation.

An advantage of the nonmodular endograft is that with a one-piece device there is no risk of late disengagement of the segments. Main disadvantages of the unibody graft are represented by the cumbersome means required for implantation, especially in the positioning of the contralateral iliac limb, and the need for extremely precise preoperative measurements. The use of this kind of endograft is still limited by the narrow spectrum of sizes available. Conversely, modular endografts are more versatile and allow assembling segments of different lengths and diameters according to the patient's anatomy. Loading catheters are usually smaller in the modular endografts, because they carry only one of the two limbs of the graft.

Endovascular Procedure

In our practice, all stent-graft procedures are carried out in the angiography suite under general anesthesia. Using a left brachial approach, a 5-F angiographic pigtail catheter is advanced into the descending aorta. This catheter allows contrast injection throughout the procedure without changing catheters through the femoral access. Routinely, mechanical injections of 25 ml nonionic contrast media with a flow of 15 ml/s are used.

For insertion of the stent graft, both common femoral arteries are surgically exposed. In case of insufficient diameter of the femoral vessels or severe calcification, the external iliac artery can be cannulated using an extraperitoneal surgical access. After achieving vascular access, 5,000 IU of heparin sodium are administered intravenously. A 5-F diagnostic multipurpose catheter is first advanced over a soft wire into the descending aorta. The wire is then exchanged for an ultrastiff guide wire (Lunderquist, Cook, 0.035" x 300 cm) to facilitate delivery of the stent graft.

TIPS AND TRICKS

A pigtail catheter placed through a brachial access into the descending aorta improves the "comfort" of the procedure by providing the ability to inject contrast at any time.

FIGURES 3A TO 3F.

Endvascular placement of a bifurcated modular stent graft for treatment of an infrarenal aortic aneurysm. (For details see text)

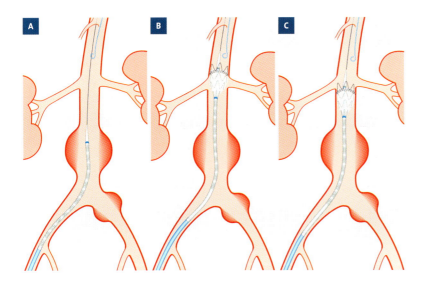

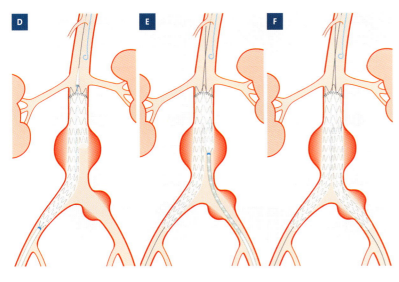

The endoprosthesis most widely used in our institution is the Talent device (Medtronic, World Medical Manufacturing Corp, Sunrise, FL, USA), which is a two-piece modular bifurcated graft consisting of an aortic main body extending into the ipsilateral iliac artery and a separate tubular graft to be used for the contralateral iliac artery. This self-expanding endoprosthesis consists of circumferential nitinol stent springs arranged as a tube for conformance to the lumen and covered on its exterior with a Dacron graft. For implantation, the Talent endoprosthesis is compressed in a PTFE sheath with an outer diameter of 24 F for the main body and 16 F for the contralateral leg. An important feature of the device are the bare springs on the top of the main body allowing suprarenal fixation.

After placement of the stiff wire, the delivery system containing the main body of the endoprosthesis is introduced through the femoral access *(Figure 3a)*. For deployment, the endoprosthesis is fixed in position with a pusher while the sheath is withdrawn. To achieve an optimal positioning of the endoprosthesis, it is advisable to start deployment of the proximal bare springs and the first covered ring slightly proximal to the renal arteries followed by contrast injection *(Figure 3b)*. After pullback of the endoprosthesis to the desired location, the rest of the endoprosthesis can be released *(Figures 3c and 3d)*. Then, a guide wire (soft angled hydrophilic guide wire, Terumo, Tokyo, Japan) is navigated from the contralateral femoral access into the connection hole "short leg" for the contralateral leg. To facilitate steerability of the guide wire, a 5-F diagnostic catheter (e.g., JR4) can be used. After achieving a correct position of the wire, the diagnostic catheter is advanced through the aortic main body, and the Terumo wire is exchanged for a stiff guide wire. The delivery device containing the contralateral leg is now advanced into the main body of the endoprosthesis and released in the same manner as described for the main body *(Figures 3e and 3f)*. A minimum overlap of two stent segments is required for fixation of the contralateral leg to the aortic part of the prosthesis. Finally, it may be helpful to use a slightly angulated projection (e.g., 25° RAO for the left leg) to ensure an optimal positioning of the contralateral leg, typically proximal to the hypogastric artery. In all cases, postdilatations of all fixation zones and the overlapping zone are performed with a compliant aortic balloon catheter (Reliant, Medtronic, World Medical Manufacturing Corp, Sunrise, FL, USA) to achieve an optimal alignment of the graft material to the vessel wall.

Postinterventional Treatment and Follow-Up

After surgical closure of the access sites, no additional anticoagulation is required. Routinely, 100 mg ASA/day is given to the patients. All patients are enrolled in a follow-up protocol including clinical examinations and follow-up CT scans before hospital discharge *(Figure 4)*, at 3 and 12 months, and yearly thereafter.

> **TIPS AND TRICKS**
>
> *In case of difficulties to navigate the wire into the connection hole for the short leg consider a transbrachial advancement of the wire together with a pull-through maneuver through the femoral sheath.*

Specific Cases (Figure 4)

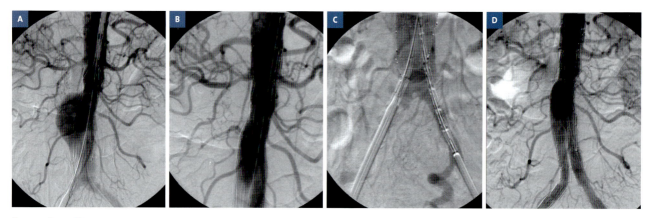

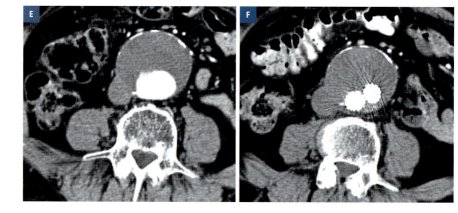

FIGURE 4A TO 4F.

Endovascular placement of a bifurcated modular stent graft (Zenith, Cook) for treatment of an infrarenal aortic aneurysm.
a) Preinterventional angio and positioning of the device.
b) Suprarenal fixation of the aortic main body with bare springs.
c) Introduction of the contralateral leg.
d) Final result.
e) Contrast-enhanced CT before and
f) 2 days after stent-graft implantation.

Summary of Outcome Results

As the prevalence and follow-up of EVAR increases, so does our understanding of the advantages and limitations of this technology. Initial clinical trials have reported high success rates for endovascular AAA exclusion, but problems detected during follow-up leave long-term durability and the effectiveness in preventing rupture of the aneurysm yet to be determined.

Studies comparing EVAR and open repair (OR) have been initially carried out in single centers in the form of case control studies, concurrent single- or multicentric prospective nonrandomized comparisons. In some instances, these studies have been used for safety and efficacy evaluation of specific endografts.

Early published series reported similar perioperative mortality rates after EVAR and OR. EVAR was associated with reduced blood loss, intensive care unit and hospital stay, and quicker recovery. These advantages came at a cost of higher local complication rates due, essentially, to graft limb and access artery problems. In the case control study by Brewster et al., the total complication rate was similar (50% with EVAR and 46% with OR), but a predominance of systemic complications in the OR group (18/28 vs. 4/28) and a prevalence of local complications in the EVAR group (16/28 vs. 2/28) were found.

Recently, May et al. reported a consecutive series of 283 patients, 135 undergoing OR and 148 EVAR. Perioperative mortality rates were not statistically different (5.9% in the OR group and 2.7% in the EVAR group), while late survival differed significantly (96% for EVAR vs. 85% for OR at 3 years). With respect to graft failure, defined in the EVAR group as exclusion of the aneurysmal sac, stability or reduction in AAA maximum transverse diameter, and persistent endoleak, the OR group had a better outcome (0 vs. 14%). The comparative report by Zarins et al. analyzed the outcome of 441 consecutive patients, 264 undergoing OR and 177 EVAR. Perioperative mortality was 3.5% and 0.5% ($p > 0.05$) for OR and EVAR groups, respectively. 4-year freedom from AAA-related death was 89% in the OR group and 95% in the EVAR group. Interestingly, incidence of secondary procedures was

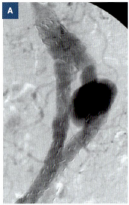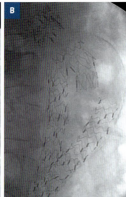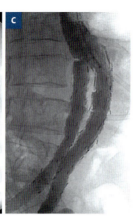

FIGURES 5A TO 5C.

Type III endoleak due to separation of the contralateral leg from the main body (a, b) treated by insertion of a stent graft (c).

not different (13% for OR vs. 15% for EVAR), but the magnitude, morbidity, and mortality of secondary procedures after OR were significantly higher.

Recently, initial results of two prospective randomized multicentric trials became available. The DREAM trial investigated EVAR vs. OR in 345 patients with AAA of at least 5 cm in diameter showing an operative mortality of 4.6% in the OR group vs. 1.2% in the EVAR group (risk ratio 3.9). The combined rate of operative mortality and severe complications was 9.8% in the OR group and 4.7% in the EVAR group, resulting in a risk ratio of 2.1.

Similar results could be obtained in the EVAR-1 trial which included a total of 1,082 patients with AAA of at least 5.5 cm diameter. 30-day mortality in the EVAR group was 1.7% vs. 4.7% in the OR group (odds ratio 0.35 [95% CI 0.16–0.77]; p = 0.009). However, data on long-term results from both trials (EVAR-1 and DREAM) showed equivalent results in both groups.

Complications of Endografting

As many of the initial patients approach the long-term follow-up period, the number of reported deficiencies associated with this technology is increasing. Some problems have been labeled as device-specific (hook fractures, modular component separation, migration), while others appear to be device-independent (endoleaks, endotension). It is also becoming clear that many patients will need secondary procedures to maintain either patency of the endograft or exclusion of the aneurysm, thus, life-long surveillance is mandatory.

Different types of failure can influence durability of EVAR.

Endoleak and Endotension

One of the principal complications after EVAR is the occurrence of "endoleak", defined as persistent blood flow outside the graft and within the aneurysmal sac. Another reason is the presence of "endotension", a state of persistent "pressurization" with consequent growth of the aneurysmal sac without evidence of extragraft blood extravasation on diagnostic imaging.

The presence of an endoleak may be due to misplacement or poor sizing of the endovascular graft (technical error) as well as to graft migration or distortion caused by material fatigue (device factors) and may be precipitated by morphologic modifications of the native vessels around the graft (patient factors).

The presence of an endoleak or endotension can expose an aneurysmal sac to systemic arterial pressure after EVAR. This persistence in pressure may be the cause of endoleak or endotension-related rupture. However, most endoleaks found in early follow-up do not lead to rupture, and not all endoleaks are predictors of mortality.

Many aspects on the nature, incidence, and significance of these problems are highly controversial. There is much controversy regarding the most appropriate diagnostic and treatment modalities for endoleaks from various endografts. Between 20% and 40% of patients undergoing EVAR experience an endoleak at some point after endograft deployment. Moreover, the real incidence of endotension is not clear, since in many cases, this finding may be due to inaccuracy of diagnostic imaging not able to show a hidden endoleak. Consequently, the detection and treatment of these phenomena have become a major consideration in endovascular surgery.

Endoleak Classification
■ Type I: seal failure

A type I endoleak comprises failure to seal the attachment sites of the endograft to the native vessels. These are widely recognized as the endoleaks most closely linked to rupture and are the most aggressively treated. Type I endoleaks can occur at proximal or distal attachment sites, and have been correlated to short aneurysm neck, large vessel diameter, aneurysm neck angulation, and tortuosity of the iliac arteries.

■ Type II: retrograde flow

As a result of retrograde flow from small arteries (such as lumbar or inferior mesenteric arteries), these can be very low-flow systems difficult to diagnose on both color duplex or CT scans. Delayed imaging may be necessary to assess late perfusion. Furthermore, interventionists debate the significance of type II endoleaks, as many of these resolve spontaneously, and the aneurysm can even shrink in the presence of such an endoleak. Early postoperative type II endoleaks can be safely observed for 6 months or longer, and treatment is based on modification of the aneurysmal sac. If the sac expands significantly during follow-up, there is little doubt that the patient should undergo treatment, usually in the form of embolization of feeding and draining vessels. More controversies exist when a type II

> **TIPS AND TRICKS**
>
> ■ *Avoid to treat short, conically shaped or severely angulated necks.*
>
> ■ *Proximal aortic necks with presence of thrombus or calcification should only be considered for EVAR if the neck is relatively long.*
>
> ■ *In case of postinterventional type II endoleaks a control CT should be performed. Only persistent endoleaks with aneurysm growth should be treated.*

endoleak is detected without a significant increase of AAA sac during follow-up. Although most of them have a benign course, cases of AAA rupture associated with type II endoleaks have been detected. Any new type II leak arising in a previously excluded aneurysmal sac should be carefully evaluated and eventually treated, as the aortic wall of a shrunken aneurysm can be less resistant to an abrupt increase of intrasac pressure.

■ Type III: graft defect

Type III endoleaks arise from a defect within the graft that can be either a disjunction between modular components (type III A) or a hole in the fabric of the graft (type III B). These endoleaks are generally graft-specific and can be serious because invariably associated with a sudden elevation of intrasac pressure potentially leading to rupture. All type III endoleaks should be repaired upon detection, using a modular extension or a covered stent or eventually with conversion to open repair.

■ Type IV: fabric porosity

Type IV endoleaks caused by fabric porosity generally subside within 30 days and do not require specific treatment.

Examples of treatment for each type of endoleak are shown in *Table 1*.

Migration

Endograft migration is an increasingly common indication for secondary intervention after EVAR. While there is discussion in the literature on the frequency and causes of migration, there is general consensus that it occurs and deserves attention. According to the Lifeline Registry reporting standards, "migration" is considered to be movement of the endograft by 5 mm or more. According to the Perugia experience, there is a cumulative migration of 27% at 3 years on 113 patients with modular, bifurcated aortic endografting. However, in this study only endografts that migrated 10 mm or more were considered. Conners et al., assuming a threshold of 5 mm for migration, found higher cumulative migration rates with the same kind of endograft: 20% at 2 years and 42% at 3 years. Overall, the incidence of distal migration ranges widely and is likely to depend on the amount of specific attention devoted to

TABLE 1.
Endoleak classification and treatment options.

Classification	Alternative definition	Opportunities for treatment
Type I	■ Graft-related	■ Proximal or distal extension or cuffs
	■ Attachment	■ Secondary endograft
	■ Perigraft	■ Open repair
Type II	■ Retrograde	■ Conservative
	■ Collateral flow	■ Coil embolization
		■ Laparoscopic clip application
		■ Intrasac injection of thrombogenic agents
Type III	■ Modular disconnection	■ Secondary endograft
	■ Fabric tear	■ Secondary endograft
Type IV	■ Porosity	■ Conservative

study the phenomenon, compliance and resolution of the imaging protocols, and size of thresholds (commonly > 10 mm or > 5 mm) to define migration. However, device, anatomic and clinical risk factors for migration have been inconsistently identified. Strategies that can reduce the risk of migration include:
- device design, with fixation mechanisms and columnar support that increases the stabilization forces;
- selection of patients with anatomy permitting long circumferential, cylindrical, sealing zones combined with optimal deployment of the graft just below the renal arteries;
- careful observations on follow-up CT scans of all modifications of the native vessels with special attention to aortic neck diameter and stent graft distance from the lowest renal artery;
- diligent patient surveillance including sensitive and frequent imaging protocols appropriate for the expected rate of migration; physician and patient must be capable and willing to reintervene prior adverse to clinical events.

The anatomic finding associated with migration that occurred most frequently was aortic neck dilatation. In the Perugia experience, a dilatation of > 3 mm occurred in 28% of the patients examined 1 year after endografting, but required reintervention only in 5.6% of the cases. Aortic neck dilatation after EVAR is a common finding also in other experiences. Other authors deny this event and hypothesize that the endograft can protect from subsequent dilatation.

Modular Component Separation

Separation of modular device components is a form of device failure that results in the rapid development of a large type III endoleak with the highest risk of AAA rupture *(Figure 5)*. The problem of limb separation is specific to the modular endograft type in which components of the stent graft are assembled in situ, as opposed to other types that are one-piece in construction. Component separation has been observed in the modular design by various manufacturers. Under nominal conditions after initial deployment of a modular stent graft, the frictional force between elements is sufficient to maintain a stable position. As the shape of the excluded aortoiliac anatomy changes in the process of shrinking, new forces are applied to the endograft. Endografts of different manufacturers may vary in their columnar strength and resistance to bending forces. Stent grafts that are relatively flexible will bend in response to the changing aorta. Stiff grafts may accumulate tension until the yielding point gives way. In some cases, this point appears to be the junction between components of the endograft. Zarins et al., in reporting seven cases of AAA rupture after EVAR, commented on the contribution of operator error in the problem of limb separation as causes of rupture. These investigators noted that early postoperative X-rays in these patients showed that the contralateral limb had been inserted into the junction between the two components for an insufficient length and, thus, was liable to separate more easily than if it had been positioned correctly.

Structural Failure

Radiographic evidence of anchoring hook fractures has been associated with insecure proximal fixation. Although hook fracture was not uniformly associated with adverse clinical consequences, Matsumura & Moore found that eight among ten explants of early EVT grafts showed attachment-system hook fractures. Most of these patients experienced graft migration with resultant endoleak that led to planned conversion; one patient survived AAA rupture.

Other examples of structural failure are the rupture of the stent, the fabric, and the suture line that supports the endograft. Unfortunately, stress tests used in mechanical bench-testing apparatus by most manufacturers to meet required testing for regulatory approval of stent graft are not comparable to the in-vivo situation primarily because they lack the variable complexity of biological systems and chaotic interactions. However, most complications associated with structural failure occurred with early endograft models that are no longer manufactured, and the impact of this problem on endografts of recent design is not yet clear.

Graft Occlusion or Stenosis

Limb occlusion or stenosis ranges widely after EVAR and generally occurs early (at approximately 3 months). The rather short time from implantation to reintervention for limb ischemia after EVAR suggests that problems with limb occlusion or stenosis are generally the result of occult iliac artery or endograft limb stenosis. A more aggressive approach to evaluating the iliac arteries reduced limb occlusion rate from 11.7% to 2.4% in Conners' experience. Furthermore, newer endograft designs have minimized this problem with more flexible supported limbs.

AAA Rupture

Prevention of rupture is, indeed, the reason for which repair is undertaken. In this regard, a recently published large series of patients treated with endovascular repair reported late rupture rates up to 1.5% per year, raising concern about durability of the procedure.

Zarins et al., reporting on 1,067 patients treated with the AneuRx endograft, found that the 1-year risk of rupture on life-table analysis was 0.4%, and the 2-year risk of rupture was 2.6%. Based on this trend, it may be reason-

> **TIPS AND TRICKS**
>
> ■ Avoid severe oversizing of the graft in the area of the iliac fixation zone because this may increase the risk of limb occlusion.

able to hypothesize that with new-generation devices and meticulous follow-up sessions concerns on rupture may become less onerous than in the past.

Vallabhaneni and Harris, reporting on patients from EUROSTAR registry, calculated a rupture rate of about 1% per year that significantly increased to 2.9% after the 5th year on life-table analysis. These results may be biased by the fact that most of the grafts with the longest follow-up are no longer in use. They also identified type III endoleak (RR 7.47), migration (RR 5.35), and aneurysm diameter at last measurement (RR 1.057) as three significant independent predictors of late rupture in the EUROSTAR population.

Although different data in the literature have reported on the risk of rupture after EVAR, it is evident that:
- second-generation aortic stent grafts appear to have better early and mid-term results,
- rigorous follow-ups of all patients after EVAR using color duplex ultrasound, plain abdominal X-ray and good-quality contrast-enhanced CT scan are crucial to avoid the disastrous consequence of rupture.

Conclusion

Endovascular grafting techniques have revolutionized the management of patients with infrarenal aneurysmal disease. However, perceived disadvantages associated with EVAR include anatomic limitations and unknown long-term durability. Early results of EVAR are comparable or superior to conventional repair. However, as patients are followed longer, various complications such as endograft disconnection, migration, and aneurysm growth or rupture have been described. Some of these problems were frequently related to early-generation endografting designs, no longer manufactured, whereas newer endografts have shown better performance although it seems early to draw definitive conclusions.

The potential dangerous consequences of complications after EVAR impose a high level of attention both preoperatively with appropriate patient selection and during follow-up with a rigorous surveillance program.

EVAR seems appropriate for high-risk patients unfit for open surgery; moreover, available evidence is competitive enough to justify the possibility of endoluminal repair in selected younger, low-risk patients. These patients should be informed of the advantages and limitations of the technique before deciding on the risks to take.

References

1. Arko FR, Lee WA, Hill BB, Olcott C, Dalman RL, Harris EJ Jr, Cipriano, Gogarty TJ, Zerins CF. Aneurysm-related death: primary endpoint analysis for comparison of open and endovascular repair. J Vasc Surg 2002;36: 297–304.

2. Becquemin J-P, d'Audiffret A, for the ACE Trialists. Abdominal aortic aneurysms – surgical versus endoluminal repair: the French prospective randomized (ACE) trial. In: Greenhalgh RM, Powell JT, Mitchell AW, eds. Vascular and endovascular opportunities. London: Saunders, 2000:234–6.

3. Beebe HG, Cronewett JL, Katzen BT, Brewster DC, Green RM, for the Vanguard Endograft Trial Investigators. Results of an aortic endograft trial: impact of device failure beyond 12 months. J Vasc Surg 2001;33:55–63.

4. Bernhard VM, Mitchell SR, Matsumura JS, Brewster DC, Decker M, Lamparello P, Raithel D, Collin J. Ruptured abdominal aortic aneurysm after endovascular repair. J Vasc Surg 2002;35:1155–62.

5. Blankensteijn JD, de Jong SE, Prinssen M, van der Ham AC, Buth J, van Sterkenburg SM, Verhagen HJ, Buskens E, Grobbee DE, Dutch Randomized Endovascular Aneurysm Management (DREAM) Trial Group. Two-year outcomes after conventional or endovascular repair of abdominal aortic aneurysms. N Engl J Med 2005;352:2398–405.

6. Brewster DC, Geller SC, Kaufman JA, Cambria RP, Gertler JP, LaMuraglia GM, Atamian S, Abbott WM. Initial experience with endovascular aneurysm repair: comparison of early results with outcome of conventional open repair. J Vasc Surg 1998;27:992–1003.

7. Buth J, Laheij RJF, for the EUROSTAR Collaborators. Early complications and endoleaks after endovascular repair of abdominal aortic aneurysm repair: report of a multicenter study. J Vasc Surg 2000;31:134–46.

8. Cao P, Verzini F, Parlani G, De Rango P, Parente B, Giordano G, Mosca S, Maselli A. Predictive factors and clinical consequences of proximal aortic neck dilatation in 230 patients undergoing AAA repair with self-expandable stent grafts. J Vasc Surg 2003;37:1200–5.

9. Cao P, Verzini F, Zannetti S, De Rango P, Parlani G, Lupattelli L, Maselli A. Device migration after endoluminal abdominal aortic aneurysm repair: analysis of 113 cases with a minimum follow-up period of 2 years. J Vasc Surg 2002;35:229–35.

10. Carpenter JP, Baum RA, Barker CF, Golden MA, Velazquez OC, Mitchell ME, Fairman RM. Durability of benefits of endovascular versus conventional abdominal aortic aneurysm repair. J Vasc Surg 2002;35:222–8.

11. Conners MS, Sternbergh WC, Carter G, Tonnessen BH, Yoselevitz M, Money SR. Endograft migration one to four years after endovascular abdominal aortic aneurysm repair with the AneuRx device: a cautionary note. J Vasc Surg 2002;36:476–84.

12. Conners MS, Sternberg WC, Carter G, Tonnessen BH, Yoselevitz M, Money SR. Secondary procedures after endovascular aortic aneurysm repair. J Vasc Surg 2002; 36:992–6.

13. Dardik A, Lin JW, Gordon TA, Williams M, Perler BA. Results of elective abdominal aortic aneurysm repair in the 1990s: a population-based analysis of 2335 cases. J Vasc Surg 1999;30:985–95.

14. EVAR Trial Participants. Endovascular aneurysm repair versus open repair in patients with abdominal aortic aneurysm (EVAR trial 1): randomised controlled trial. Lancet 2005; 365:2179–86.

15. Faries PL, Brener BJ, Connelly TL, Katzen BT, Briggs VL, Burks JA Jr, Gravereaux EC, Carrocio A, Morrissey NJ, Toedorescu V, Won J, Sparacino S, Chae KS, Hollier LH, Marin ML. A multicenter experience with Talent endovascular graft for the treatment of abdominal aortic aneurysm. J Vasc Surg 2002;35:1123–8.

16. Greenberg RK, Ouriel K, Shortell C, Green RM, Sunita D, Srivastava SD, Waldman D, Iling KA, Ivancev K. An endoluminal method of hemorrhage control and repair of ruptured abdominal aortic aneurysms. J Endovasc Ther 2000;7:1–7.

17. Greenhalgh RM, Brown LC, Kwong GP, Powell JT, Thompson SG; EVAR trial participants. Comparison of endovascular aneurysm repair with open repair in patients with abdominal aortic aneurysm (EVAR trial 1), 30-day operative mortality results: randomised controlled trial. Lancet 2004;364:843–8.

18. Greenhalgh RM, Brown LC,Powell JT, for the UK EVAR Trial Participants. The UK EndoVascular Aneurysm Repair (EVAR) trials: background and methodology. In: Greenhalgh RM, Powell JT, Mitchell AW, eds. Vascular and endovascular opportunities. London: Saunders, 2000:215–27.

19. Hinchliffe RJ, Yusuf SW, Macierewicz JA, MacSweeney STR, Wenham PW, Hopkinson BR. Endovascular repair of ruptured abdominal aortic aneurysm – a challenge to open repair? Results of a single center experience in 20 patients. Eur J Vasc Endovasc Surg 2001;22:528–34.

20. Jacobowitz GR, Lee AM, Riles TS. Immediate and late explantation of endovascular aortic grafts: the endovascular technologies experience. J Vasc Surg 1999;29:309–16.

21. Laheij RJ, Buth J, Harris PL, Moll FL, Stelter WJ, Verhoeven EL. Need for secondary interventions after endovascular repair of abdominal aortic aneurysms. Intermediate-term follow-up results of a European collaborative registry (EUROSTAR). Br J Surg 2000; 87:1666–73.

22. Lifeline Registry of Endovascular Aneurysm Repair Steering Committee. Lifeline registry: collaborative evaluation of endovascular aneurysm repair. J Vasc Surg 2001;34:1139–46.

23. Makaroun MS, Chaikof E, Naslund T, Matsumura JS, for the EVT Investigators. Efficacy of a bifurcated endograft versus open repair of abdominal aortic aneurysms: a reappraisal. J Vasc Surg 2002;35:203–10.

24. Makaroun MS, Deaton D. Is proximal aortic neck dilatation after endovascular aneurysm exclusion a cause of concern? J Vasc Surg 2001;35:S39–45.

25. Matsumura JK, Chaikof EL, for the EVT Investigators. Continued expansion of aortic necks after endovascular repair of abdominal aortic aneurysms. J Vasc Surg 1998;28:422–31.

26. Matsumura JS, Moore WS, for the Endovascular Technologies Investigators. Clinical consequences of peroprosthetic leak after endovascular repair of abdominal aortic aneurysms. J Vasc Surg 1998;27:606–13.

27. May J, White GH, Ly CN, Jones MA, Harris JP. Endoluminal repair of abdominal aortic aneurysm prevents enlargement of the proximal neck: a 9-year lifetable and 5-year longitudinal study. J Vasc Surg 2003; 37:86–90.

28. May J, White GH, Waugh R, Ly CN, Stephen MS, Jones MA, Harris JP. Improved survival after endoluminal repair with second-generation prostheses compared with open repair in the treatment of abdominal aortic aneurysms: a 5-year concurrent comparison using life table method. J Vasc Surg 2001;33:S21–6.

29. May J, White GH, Waugh R, Petrasek P, Chaufour X, Arulchelvam M, Stephen MS, Harris JP. Life-table analysis of primary and assisted success following endoluminal repair of abdominal aortic aneurysms: the role of supplementary endovascular intervention in improving outcome. Eur J Vasc Endovasc Surg 2000; 19:648–55.

30. Okhi T, Veith FJ, Sanchez LA, Cynamon J, Lipsitz EC, Wain RA, Morgan JA, Zhen L, Suggs WD, Lyon RT. Endovascular graft repair of ruptured aortoiliac aneurysms. J Am Coll Surg 1999;189:102–12.

31. Parlani G, Zannetti S, Verzini F, De Rango P, Carlini G, Lenti M, Cao P. Does the presence of an iliac aneurysm affect outcome of endoluminal AAA Repair? An analysis of 336 cases. Eur J Vasc Endovasc Surg 2002;24:134–8.

32. Politz JK, Newman VS, Stewart MT. Late abdominal aortic aneurysm rupture after AneuRx repair: a report of three cases. J Vasc Surg 2000;31:599–606.

33. Prinssen M, Buskens E, Blankesteijn JD. The Dutch Randomised Endovascular Aneurysm Management (DREAM) trial. J Cardiovasc Surg 2002;43:379–84.

34. Prinssen M, Verhoeven EL, Buth J, Cuypers PW, van Sambeek MR, Balm R, Buskens E, Grobbee DE, Blankesteijn JD, Dutch Randomized Endovascular Aneurysm Management (DREAM) Trial Group. A randomized trial comparing conventional and endovascular repair of abdominal aortic aneurysms. N Engl J Med 2004;351:1607–18.

35. Q1 2002 EVEM Panel Report. EVEM online: Vascularnews.com/evem/index.htm; zainab@bibamedical.com.

36. Vallabhaneni R, Harris P. Overview of the complications following endovascular AAA repair. In: Brancherau A, Jacobs M, Eds. Complications in vascular and endovascular surgery, part II. Armonk: Blackwell Publishing, 2002:129–36.

37. Veith FJ, Baum RA, Ohki T, Amor M, Adiseshiah M, Blankesteijn JD, Buth J, Chuter TA, Fairman RM, Gilling-Smith G, Harris PL, Hodgson KJ, Hopkinson BR, Ivancev K, Katzen BT, Lawrence-Brown M, Meier GH, Malina M, Makaroun MS, Parodi JC, Richter GM, Rubin GD, Stelter WJ, White GH, White RA, Wisselink W, Zarins CK. Nature and significance of endoleaks and endotension: summary of opinions expressed at an international conference. J Vasc Surg 2002;35:1029–35.

38. Wever JJ, Nie AJ de, Blankesteijn JD, Broeders IAMJ, Mali WPTM, Eikelboom BC. Dilatation of the proximal neck of infrarenal aortic aneurysms after endovascular AAA repair. Eur J Vasc Endovasc Surg 2000; 19:197–201.

39. Yusuf SW, Whitaker SC, Chuter TA, Wenham PW, Hopkinson BR. Emergency endovascular repair of leaking aortic aneurysm. Lancet 1994;344:1645–50.

40. Zarins CK, Arko FR, Lee WA, Hill BB, Olcott C, Dalman RL, et al. Effectiveness of endovascular versus open repair in prevention of aneurysm related death. Proceedings of the 49th Scientific Meeting of the American Association for Vascular Surgery, Baltimore, June 2001.

41. Zarins CK, White RA, Fogarty TJ. Aneurysm rupture after endovascular repair using the AneuRx stent graft. J Vasc Surg 2000;31:960–70.

42. Zarins CK, White RA, Hodgson KJ, for the AneuRx Clinical Investigators. Endoleak as a predictor of outcome following endovascular aneurysm repair. AneuRx Multicenter Clinical Trial. J Vasc Surg 2000;32:90–107.

43. Zarins CK, White RA, Moll FL, Crabtree T, Bloch DA, Hodgson KJ. The AneuRx stent graft: four-year results and worldwide experience. J Vasc Surg 2000;33:S135–45.

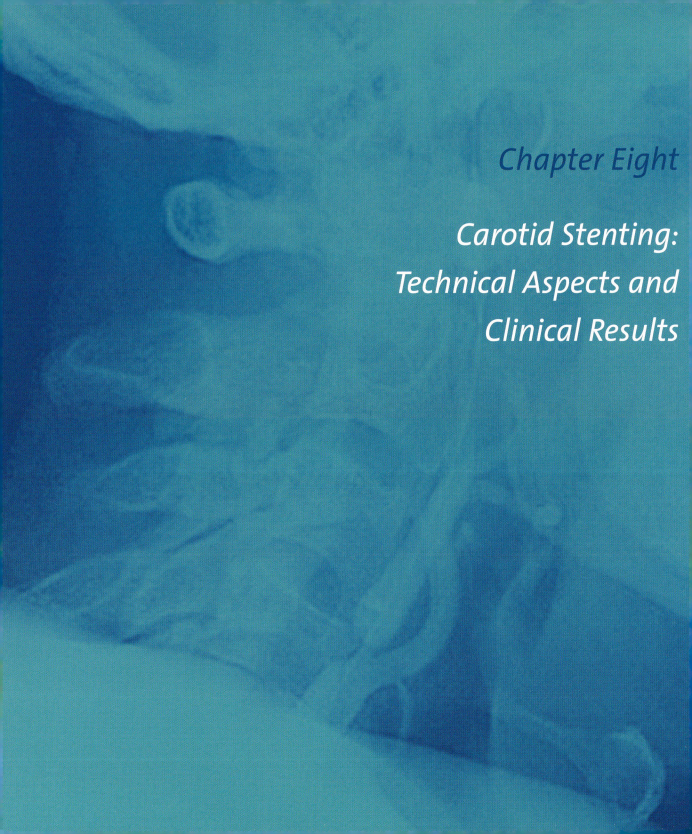

Chapter Eight

Carotid Stenting: Technical Aspects and Clinical Results

Introduction

Endovascular carotid stenting is an evolving technology offering an alternative to carotid endarterectomy (CEA) for treatment of carotid stenosis.

Carotid artery stenting (CAS) is probably a less invasive and less traumatic means of achieving the goal of prevention of embolization of plaque material or occlusion of the related internal carotid artery (ICA).

The efficacy of CAS depends on the ability of the interventionalists to produce a complication-free result. This can only be achieved after a dedicated and intensive training period as well as by careful attention to the patient selection and technical details.

During the last few years there have been dramatic changes in the technique of CAS, driven largely by the introduction of smaller stent delivery systems and new stents.

In particular the application of "neuroprotection devices" specifically designed to avoid embolization of debris released during the different steps of the stenting procedure has added an important new dimension to the performance of a safe CAS.

Finally, it is increasingly evident that experienced interventionalists are able to perform CAS with acute and long-term outcomes that compare favorably with CEA in high-risk patients, and probably also in asymptomatic patients showing relevant stenotic disease of the ICA.

CONTENTS DVD

15. Recanalization of left subclavian artery occlusion (09:35 min)
16. Carotid artery stenting with filter protection (12:12 min)
17. Carotid artery stenting with proximal protection (14:23 min)

Evaluation of the Patient

A complete history and examination are essential before considering a carotid intervention. We have to keep in mind that in the majority of the cases we have to deal with polymorbid patients showing, in at least 55% of the cases, a relevant coronary heart disease (CHD) or more often a peripheral arterial occlusive disease (PAOD).

Furthermore, many patients referred for treatment of carotid stenosis manifest neurologic symptoms related to other causes, so that CAS will not resolve their problems. Particularly in patients with preexisting deficits it is essential to have a neurologic evaluation prior to considering any type of intervention.

To evaluate the indication of the procedure, an MRA/CT angio and a carotid duplex scan are mandatory. The final decision for an intervention will be taken after the preinterventional angiography confirming the noninvasive evaluation.

In fact, in our experience the validity of the color-coded Doppler is very technician-dependent and can either overestimate or underestimate the severity of the lesion.

MRAs tend, in many cases, to overestimate the degree of stenosis and pretend an interpretation with caution. Because of that, in our experience, only the combination of the findings may permit a relatively consistent diagnosis.

> **TIPS AND TRICKS**
>
> - *Only symptomatic stenoses of > 70% or asymptomatic stenoses of the ICA > 80% should be considered for intervention.*

Vascular Access

For CAS the transfemoral approach is strongly preferred.

In patients with severely diseased pelvic arteries or an extremely elongated aorta, the transbrachial or radial access may be an alternative. The right carotid should be accessed via the left brachial and vice versa.

The common carotid artery (CCA) is normally cannulated with a right Judkins catheter or with a mammaria catheter (Bernstein or Vertebralis are an alternative). In some cases a Sidewinder or Vitek catheter may be necessary. After entering the target vessel a guide wire with a hydrophilic coating is advanced into the CCA or ECA (external carotid artery). Over this wire a long 6-F is introduced. Direct carotid puncture has been performed in the past in specific anatomic situations such as very tortuous arteries or occluded arteries preventing a standard access. Direct CCA puncture has a markedly higher risk of complications, e.g. carotid dissection, carotid thrombosis while achieving hemostasis after sheath removal, or airway compromise from hematoma.

Diagnostic Catheter Techniques

The aortic arch anatomy is determining the approach used for cannulation of the target vessel. In this context, a classification of the aortic arch into types I – III has been proposed *(Figure 1)*.

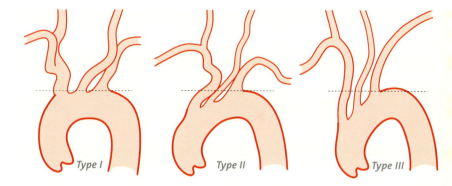

FIGURE 1. Anatomic differences of the aortic arch.

When all of the great vessels originate at the same level as a line drawn from the origin of the left subclavian artery, the arch is classified as type I and carotid access is relatively straightforward. If the origins of the innominate or the left CCA are markedly inferiorly displaced relative to this line, the arch is classified as type II or type III and access is more difficult since a catheter approaching from the descending aorta will tend to prolapse into the ascending aorta as it is pushed into these deep-seated arteries.

To visualize the origin of the arch vessels an angiogram via pigtail catheter (30° LAO) should be routinely performed before choosing the adequate catheter for the selective cannulation of the CCA.

The catheter is gently pulled back until it slips into the brachiocephalic trunk. Thereafter, the hydrophilic wire is advanced into the right CCA. Keeping the wire in position, the catheter is advanced using a "pull-and-push technique" into the CCA *(Figure 2c)*.

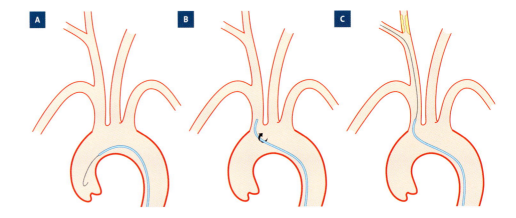

FIGURES 2A TO 2C.
Cannulation of the supraaortic vessels in case of normal aortic arch configuration.

In our institution to cannulate the CCA in type I or II arch, routinely, a 5-F diagnostic catheter (right Judkins) is advanced over a 0.035" glide wire into the ascending aorta *(Figure 2)*.

When placed in the lower aortic arch, the tip of the catheter should point inferiorly or be placed over a guide wire. This forestalls traumatic lesions of the intima of the aortic arch and prevents the catheter from being trapped in vessel ostia. Also, the wire can be used to stiffen the catheter *(Figure 2a)*.

When reaching the ascending aorta, the catheter is turned around 180°, which places the tip in an upright position *(Figure 2b)*.

To enter the left CCA the catheter is pulled back very slowly from the ostium of the brachiocephalic trunk. It should be turned 20° counterclockwise to have the tip of the catheter pointing slightly anteriorly. In elongated aortic arches, the origin of the left CCA migrates posteriorly. In this case the catheter may have to be rotated posteriorly instead of anteriorly.

The position of the catheter can be confirmed through a small injection of contrast agent. After engaging the left CCA the catheter should be turned 20° clockwise to point the tip vertically or slightly posteriorly again. Thereafter, the hydrophilic wire is advanced up to the distal CCA, followed by the catheter.

> **TIPS AND TRICKS**
>
> ■ *Injections of contrast agents in all brachiocephalic arteries should be performed by hand and with only small amounts of agent (no more than 6 cm^3 per injection).*

More complex vessel anatomy may impose to switch to Vitek or Simmons/Sidewinder or Mani catheters. After forming a loop in the ascending aorta *(Figure 3a)*, these catheters have to be gently pulled back under rotation to slip into the vessels of the aortic arch.

The wire is always used to enter the artery first, followed by the catheter. *(Figure 3b)* The advancement of the catheter is performed slowly. At the same time the wire is withdrawn, so it should not change the position. The advancement of the catheter and withdrawal of the wire are performed alternately as long as the catheter is placed securely in the CCA.

This technique using a Simmons-catheter is also applied if a brachial access is chosen *(Figure 4a and 4b)*. A right brachial approach is used for a left carotid stenosis, a left brachial access is chosen for PTA of a right carotid stenosis.

There are several reasons why advancement of the catheter into the carotid artery may be very difficult.

If the wire is not strong enough to support the catheter, it should be placed further distally or be exchanged to a stiffer wire.

Particularly in case of an angulated origin of the left CCA, the advancement of a catheter is only possible if the glide wire is kept in a firm position. In these cases, we recommend to navigate

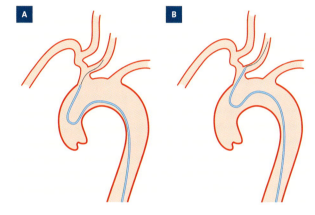

FIGURES 3A AND 3B.
Cannulation of the left CCA in case of complex aortic arch anatomy.

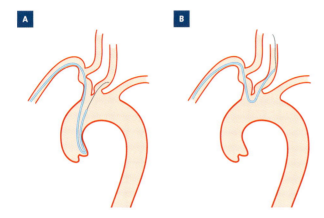

FIGURES 4A AND 4B.

Transbrachial approach. Cannulation of the left CCA using a Simmons catheter via a right brachial access.

the glide wire into the ECA first before advancing the diagnostic catheter.

A sharp angle at the distal end of the catheter due to vessel kinkings can be reduced by rotating the catheter gently while holding the wire fixed, until the catheter can be placed at the desired position.

If the advancement is still unsuccessful, a Simmons III catheter may be necessary to advance the glide wire into the ECA. Eventually, torqueing of the wire might help advancing. Then, the Simmons III catheter can be exchanged with a multipurpose catheter (4 or 5 F).

In some cases to enter the left ECA the patient's head should be turned to the contralateral side and be flexed to separate the ECA from the ICA and to align the ICA with the CCA. The tip of the catheter should point posteriorly.

Several other approaches are useful and the operator should be familiar with these techniques.

> **TIPS AND TRICKS**
>
> ■ *The Telescoping technique is highly successful for placement of a sheath or guiding catheter into the CCA.*

One relatively often used approach that works well with different anatomies, is the telescoping access technique, prepared with a 125-cm JR4 or Vitek catheter inserted through a 6-F 90 cm long Cook Shuttle sheath (Cook Inc., Bloomington, IN, USA) or an 8-F H1 guide (Cordis Incorporated, Miami Lakes, FL, USA). A stiff-angled 0.035" glide wire (Terumo Inc. Somerset, NJ, USA) is passed through the diagnostic catheter.

The diagnostic catheter is used to engage the innominate or left CCA. The ECA and ICA should be adequately separated in an optimal view.

If possible, a PA or LAO view should be used so that the sheath/guide catheter movement in the aortic arch is adequately visualized. The RAO views are often better for opening up the right carotid bifurcation, but in this view it is difficult to assess the behavior of the sheath or guide catheter in the aortic arch.

Once a road map is obtained through the diagnostic catheter, the stiff-angled glide wire is advanced through the diagnostic catheter into the ECA and then the diagnostic catheter is advanced into the mid CCA over the glide wire. The glide wire and diagnostic catheter are then used as a rail to advance the sheath or guiding catheter into the mid CCA.

Small rotational movements of the sheath are helpful in atraumatic advancement of the sheath. When a guide catheter is used, a small counter-clockwise rotation is often helpful in seating the guide catheter into the CCA.

At this point, the diagnostic catheter and glide wire can be withdrawn with some countertraction applied to the guide catheter or sheath since occasionally, it will tend to jump forward as the diagnostic catheter and glide wire are withdrawn. The guide catheter or sheath should be allowed to bleed back at this point so as to wash out any debris that may have collected at the tip during the advancement of the system to the CCA.

With experience and if the arch is friendly (type I or II), a coronary approach can be used and the CCA can be engaged directly with an H1 guide catheter.

In experienced hands, this approach is safe and faster than the other approaches. In a bovine arch where the left CCA originates from the innominate, it is often faster to use an AL1 guide to engage the ostium and proximal left CCA. This approach is particularly helpful when a bovine takeoff is combined with severe CCA disease or occlusion of the ECA so that it is not possible to put a 0.035" wire very far into the left CCA. With this technique, it is occasionally necessary to place a stiff 0.014" or 0.018" wire in the CCA or ECA to maintain guide stability.

In the presence of severe disease of the CCA ostium, the telescoping approach should not be used, since the small gap between the diagnostic catheter and sheath edge may cause plaque dissection or embolization. The sheath should be advanced over the dilator to minimize trauma. With very severe ostial disease, it is necessary to treat the ostium first before proceeding to the ICA.

> **TIPS AND TRICKS**
>
> *In a bovine arch the AL1, EBU or Simmons II guiding catheter should only engage the ostium of the left CCA.*

Angiography

For comparison before versus after carotid stenting and to be prepared for further intracranial rescue procedures in case of embolization, it is mandatory to perform an intracranial angiography in two projections, lateral and AP-30° cranial.

Carotid Sheath/Guiding Catheter Placement

Using the technique favored in our center, before exchanging the diagnostic 5-F catheter for an introducer sheath, it is necessary to cannulate the ECA. Many investigators recommend a road mapping to display the origin of the ECA. To use bony landmarks, is an alternative.

After engaging the ECA with a glide wire and placement of the diagnostic catheter in a firm position, the glide wire is exchanged with a long 0.035" stiff wire (300 cm) which can safely be placed in a distal branch of the ECA (Super-stiff Amplatz, Cook or Supracore, Guidant).

The diagnostic catheter is removed keeping the position of the superstiff wire constant in the distal ECA. Over the wire a 6- to 7-F 90-cm preflushed vascular sheath (Arrow, Cook or Terumo) or the corresponding guiding catheter (8 F) is then advanced into the CCA proximal to the bifurcation.

With the use of distal filter protection devices it is critical that the operator always be aware of the position of the guiding catheter. In consequence, the use of a lateral view is not recommended, because in the lateral view the guide catheter or sheath in the CCA is generally not visible. With distal protection in place, prolapse of the guide catheter into the aortic arch could lead to the withdrawal of the deployed system through the lesion, which could result in ICA dissection or a stroke. Therefore, when using a filter we prefer to work in an ipsilateral oblique view, which allows visualization of the lesion, as well as visualization of the CCA so that we can monitor the position of the guiding catheter within this artery.

Sheath versus Guiding Catheter

The use of a long sheath versus a guiding catheter is a matter of operator preference, and there are benefits and disadvantages to each approach. Our practice had been to use the 90-cm sheaths, but in some cases we have found the torqueability of guiding catheters to be helpful in both placing the distal filter as well as the capture sheaths needed for retrieving the filter after stenting.

In addition, if the guiding catheter starts sliding out of the CCA, it is often possible to maneuver it upward again, but this is generally not possible when a sheath prolapses out of the CCA. Finally, in cases with extreme tortuosity in the proximal left CCA, it is possible to use an angulated guide (Hockey stick) to engage the ostium of the CCA and perform the carotid stenting procedure without having to traverse the CCA.

The Stenting Procedure

The first step consists in the placement of the sheath or guiding catheter in the CCA and selection of the opportune neuroprotection system (NPS).

Using an endovascular clamping, the lesion will be passed with a conventional guide wire of choice already under effective protection. By contrast, the passage of the lesion with a distal protection system will occur without protection. Rarely, a completely unprotected predilatation is needed to introduce a filter device.

During the procedure the heart rate and the blood pressure have to be monitored continuously. We try to avoid any type of sedation with the clear intention to continously control the reaction of the patient asking her/him to speak and move the contralateral hand and/or leg.

An independent neurologic examination, including the National Institutes of Health Stroke Scale should be performed before and after all procedures.

Predilatation

Predilatation after placement of the protection system is performed to facilitate the delivery of the stent in severe stenosis. Some investigators perform it routinely, in our center we prefer to use it only when the degree of stenosis and/or a severe calcifications may prevent direct stenting.

For predilatation a 2.5- or 3.0-mm monorail coronary angioplasty balloon is used. To minimize the potential liberation of debris, it is normally inflated at low pressure and just for few seconds.

Embolic Protection Devices

Despite all the great technological improvements, the use of antecedent and periprocedural antiplatelet therapies, including heparinization, the "pending sword of Damocles" of CAS remains to be – also for the experienced interventionalist – the unpredictable embolic neurologic event caused by debris of the obstructing plaque, containing friable and sclerotic material combined with thrombotic appositions.

The daily clinical experience indicates that the composition of the obstructive plaque, estimated by different techniques such as ultrasound, MRA, spiral CT, or angiography in the majority of the cases cannot predict the quantity or quality of potentially deleterious debris.

To minimize the risk of embolic events, several protection strategies have been proposed and partially extensively used in the clinical routine.

In fact, at least in 60% of the cases debris were captured during the procedure using any type of protection device.

At present, three different concepts of neuroprotection have been introduced and clinically evaluated: distal occlusion balloon, distal filters, and proximal endovascular clamping.

Distal Occlusion of the ICA Using the Percusurge Guard Wire™ (Medtronic, Minneapolis, MN, USA)

The Guard Wire™ was the first neuroprotection device available on the market. The occlusion balloon is fixed on the tip of a guide wire (0.014" or 0.018"; *Figure 5*).

After evacuation, the balloon (4.0 – 6.0 mm) can be filled with a saline/contrast agent mixture connecting the wire to the so-called Micro-Seal™ adapter. After placement of a guiding catheter (8 F) or long sheath (6–7 F) in the corresponding CCA, the Guard Wire™

> **TIPS AND TRICKS**
>
> Although there are still some interventionalists who would prefer to protect the patient against protection devices rather than the brain against emboli, we would like to assert that CAS without neuroprotection is not ethically acceptable anymore.

FIGURE 5.
Distal balloon protection with Percusurge system.

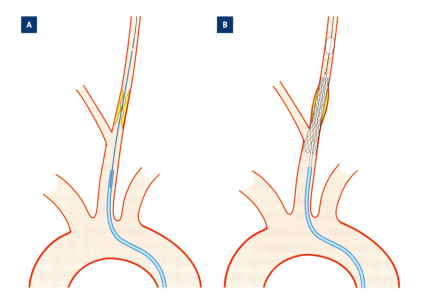

is navigated through the lesion. Before inflation, the balloon should be positioned 3.5 – 4.0 cm distal to the lesion.

After controlling the effectivity of the distal flow blockage by gently injecting a few milliliters of contrast, the Micro Seal™ is closed and removed.

The Guard Wire™ (190 or 300 cm) is thereafter used as a conventional guide wire for the subsequent stenting procedure.

After stent postdilatation the third part of the system (the Expert™ catheter) is advanced over the Guard Wire™ through the stent toward the still blocking balloon, before starting to aspirate blood including the liberated debris (20-cm^3 syringe).

Normally, the amount of aspirated blood is 60 – 100 ml; if necessary more, finally permitting to capture also very small particles *(Example 1)*.

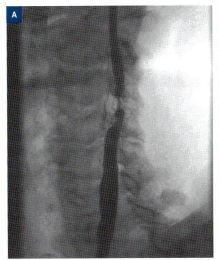
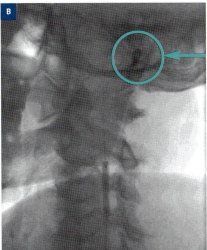
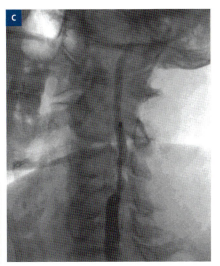
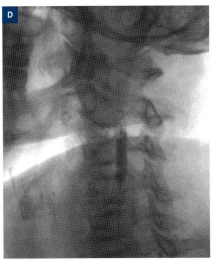
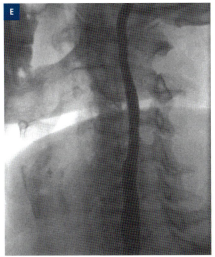

EXAMPLES 1A TO 1E.

a) High-grade stenosis left ICA, occlusion of the ECA.
b) Inflated occlusion balloon for endovascular clamping of the ICA.
c) Positioning of a self-expanding stent in the ICA stenosis.
d) Postdilatation of the stent.
e) Final angiography after declamping of the ICA.

An advantage of this technique is the very low crossing profile of the Guard Wire™ (2.7 F).

Disadvantages include the relative complexity of the system, as well as the impossibility of an angiographic control during the procedure. More important, however, is the fact that in 10 – 15% of the procedures a neurologic intolerance to the flow blockage may occur.

In such cases, it is often possible to conclude the procedure with stepwise aspiration of blood, deflation of the balloon with restoration of antegrade blood flow and, finally, after an adequate recovery time, reblockage of the ICA. Of

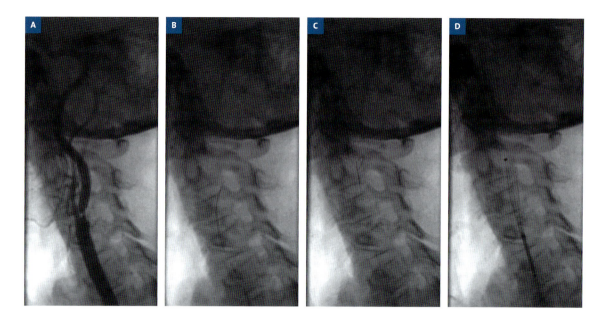

EXAMPLES 2A TO 2D.
a) High-grade stenosis left ICA.
b) After introduction of a 6-F/90-cm sheath passage of the stenosis with a Filterwire EZ™ (Boston Scientific).
c) Opening of the filter in the distal ICA.
d) Deployment of a selfexpanding stent in the ICA stenosis.

course, this type of complication may prolong the stenting procedure significantly, potentially increasing the periprocedural complication rate.

The clinical introduction of distal filter devices has ousted this technique from many centers in Europe.

Filter Systems

During the last few years, different filter devices have been proposed and clinically tested. One of the advantages of the filters over the distal occlusive balloon system is the maintenance of blood flow throughout the procedure increasing the tolerance for a safe CAS procedure.

In principle, all filters are mounted on the shaft of a guide wire (0.014"). To avoid an opening of the system before correct placement has been achieved, all filters have to be premounted on or introduced in a delivery catheter.

After preshaping the soft distal tip of the guide wire, the protection system (2.7 – 4.1 F) is passed through the target

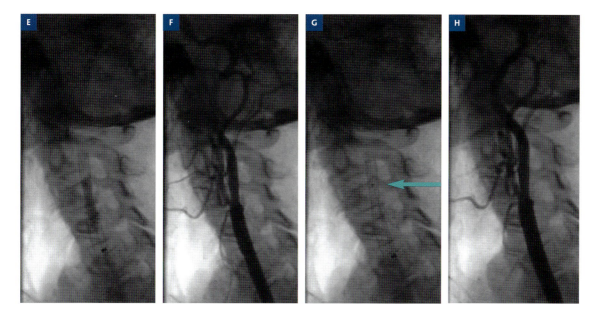

lesion *(Examples 2a, b)*, if possible using the road-map technique.

This step of the procedure and the following release of the filter, withdrawing the delivery catheter *(Example 2c)*, are an unprotected step of the procedure and in ~ 1% may be related to neurologic complications.

The filters have to be placed in a straight segment (landing zone) to optimize the adaptation of the frame to the vessel wall at least 3–4 cm distal of the lesion.

In front of very tight calcified stenoses it may be impossible to navigate the system into the ICA.

A risky unprotected predilatation using conventional coronary techniques is then necessary before filter placement. With the improvement of the steerability and torqueability of the new generation of filter devices, the need for such manipulations or the use of "buddy wires" could be relevantly reduced.

Before starting the stenting procedure *(Example 2d)* it is mandatory to control the stable and optimal position of the filter by injecting contrast agent. It is very important to stress the fact, that to maintain the same position of the filter throughout the different steps of the procedure is not trivial, but of utmost importance to avoid spasms of the very reactive ICA.

Finally, after delivery and postdilatation of the stent each filter has to be gently recaptured with a dedicated retrieval catheter *(Examples 2e–h)*.

Filter devices can be separated in two groups. Either the filter is pre-

EXAMPLE 2E TO 2H.

e) *Postdilatation of the stent.*
f) *Angiographic control after postdilatation and before retrieval of the filter.*
g) *Introduction of a catheter for retrieval of the filter (arrow).*
h) *Final angiographic result.*

mounted on the shaft of the guide wire or the lesion is first crossed with a guide wire and thereafter the filter is deployed using a separate delivery catheter. The second concept requires an additional step during the intervention, however, a guide wire of choice can be used, which might be an advantage in case of difficult lesions.

Premounted filter systems are, for example, the Filterwire EZ™ (Boston Scientific Corp., Natick, MA, USA), which was used in the BEACH trial, the Angioguard XP™ (Cordis, Miami Lakes, FL, USA) used in the SAPPHIRE trial, and the ACCUNET™ Embolic Protection Device (Guidant, Indianapolis, IN, USA) tested and validated in the ARCHER trials I–III. Some filters are available in different sizes (Angioguard XP™, ACCUNET™), other designs allow the application of one size for different vessel diameters (Filterwire EZ™).

Using the SpideRX™ (ev3, Plymouth, MN, USA) or the Emboshield® (MedNova, Abbott, Abbott Place, IL, USA) validated in the SECURITY study, first the lesion is passed with a guide wire and thereafter the filter is delivered via a separate catheter.

The Rubicon Filter (Rubicon, Salt Lake City, UT, USA) has a unique design and is the only filter without a dedicated delivery catheter. Therefore, it has a very low profile of 2.0–2.4 F. The filter is deployed via a coaxial actuating wire at the proximal end of the guide wire.

Endovascular clamping

PARODI AES (ArteriA medical Science, San Francisco, CA, USA)

This device prevents distal embolization by establishing a retrograde flow in the ICA. It consists of a 10-F guiding catheter with an integrated balloon at its distal tip. This balloon is inflated in the CCA. To avoid retrograde blood flow from the ECA to the ICA the former is occluded with a separate balloon mounted on a wire which is introduced through the 7-F lumen of the guiding catheter. The proximal hub of the guiding catheter is connected with a venous sheath. Due to the pressure difference between the distal ICA and the venous system a retrograde blood flow is established. A filter located in the arteriovenous shunt prevents embolization of the debris into the venous system.

One advantage of this technique is that because of the flow reversal during the procedure emboli cannot move toward the brain. The protection starts already before crossing the lesion. A disadvantage is the intolerance of balloon occlusion in some patients.

Mo.Ma™ Neuroprotection Device (Invatec s.r.l., Roncadelle, Italy)

The Mo.Ma device is a single-catheter system that integrates the functional aspects of a cerebral protection device and a shuttle sheath with a 6-F working channel to perform stent implantation and for the removal of particulate debris by aspiration. The system permits endovascular clamping of both the CCA (maximum diameter 13 mm) and the ECA (maximum diameter 7 mm) via two independently inflatable low-pressure compliant balloons. Blood flow of the carotid arteries is blocked during the procedure, before a guide wire or other devices are advanced across the lesion. Dislodged material can be removed intermittently between the single steps or at the end of the procedure by aspiration of blood through the working channel.

CAS Procedure Using the Mo.Ma System (Figure 6)

After inserting a 9-F/25-cm introducer sheath through the common femoral artery (CFA) into the aorta, a diagnostic angiography of the supra-aortic vessels is performed and the carotid artery to be treated is selectively displayed. Using a "push-and-pull" technique, the diagnostic catheter is then inserted into the ECA over a soft 0.035" hydrophilic-coated guide wire *(Figure 6a)*. Once the diagnostic catheter is inside the ECA, the soft guide wire can be easily exchanged with a high-support 250–300 cm long 0.035" wire *(Figure 6b)*. After withdrawing the diagnostic catheter, the Mo.Ma system can be inserted via the stiff wire into the ECA and the CCA *(Figure 6c)*. Once correct positioning and orientation of the device have been confirmed by angiography, the distal (ECA) balloon is inflated and the guide wire removed. After inflating the proximal (CCA) balloon *(Figure 6d)*, the effectiveness of antegrade blood flow interruption must be checked by slowly injecting a small (2–3 cm^3) amount of contrast medium and by verifying that contrast stagnation occurs at the carotid bifurcation. Contrast medium is then reaspirated. At the same time, patient tolerance to endovascular clamping must be clinically controlled. Immediately afterwards, treatment of the carotid lesion can be carried out conventionally *(Figures 6e–h)*. After deploying the stent and subsequent dilatation, multiple syringe blood aspirations must be performed via the proximal lateral port of the Mo.Ma system in order to remove any particles *(Figure 6i)*. Blood aspirated by syringe must be filtered in the sterile field. After no more particulate debris appears in the filter, the balloons can be deflated and the Mo.Ma system removed via the introducer sheath *(Figure 6j; Example 3)*.

Monitoring of the "back pressure" (the blood pressure measured at the carotid bifurcation during clamping of CCA and ECA) has shown to serve as an adjunctive parameter, which may be very useful to assess or predict patient tolerance to antegrade blood flow blockage. Stable values of > 30 mmHg have been shown to predict good patient tolerance.

The Mo.Ma system has been evaluated in the European Registry (157 patients in 14 centers).

In all patient the device was successfully positioned and a stent implanted. The mean duration of flow blockage was 7.6 min. In hospital, two minor strokes (2.6%), but no major stroke or death were observed.

These results have been confirmed by the "Priamus" registry including 416 patients in four Italian centers.

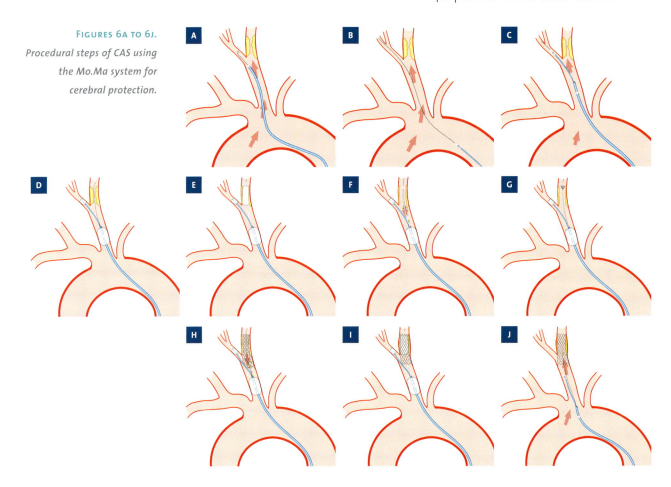

FIGURES 6A TO 6J.
Procedural steps of CAS using the Mo.Ma system for cerebral protection.

Carotid Stenting: Technical Aspects and Clinical Results

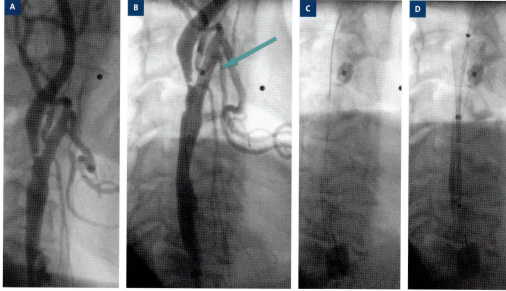

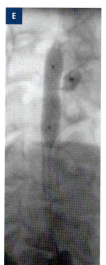

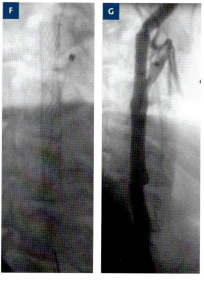

EXAMPLES 3A TO 3G.
a) High grade stenosis right ICA.
b) Positioning of the Mo.Ma system with the marker of the distal balloon for clamping the ECA in the proximal ECA (arrow).
c) After endovascular clamping of the CCA and ECA, passage of the ICA stenosis with a guide wire.
d) Deployment of a self-expanding stent in the ICA stenosis.
e) Postdilatation of the stent.
f) After aspiration of potential debris declamping of the ECA and CCA balloon.
g) Final angiogram.

Comments

One major issue presenting the different types of neuroprotection devices is related to the fact that the technology is continuously and rapidly evolving, precluding, in consequence, the possibility to give a final judgment of the systems.

In fact, depending on the different stages of development, testing, approval or clearance of a device, study results are often presented later than the "new" generation.

This fact is valid particularly for the filter devices: the BEACH, SAPPHIRE, SECURITY, and ARCHER trials are reporting results obtained with an antecedent generation of filters.

Furthermore, the present study situation does not permit to express a comparative evaluation of the different systems.

A head-to-head comparison of the different filter devices is unrealistic, because in experienced hands the CAS procedure-related complication rate is so low that it will be difficult to perform studies with adequate power to compare the efficacy and to demonstrate the superiority of a filter system.

Nevertheless, recent studies have clearly demonstrated, in an "in vitro" model focusing on carotid anatomy, that not all filters are equally effective and most significantly none of the four tested filters prevented embolization completely.

On the other hand, the clinical importance of cerebral microemboli remains controversial, as no clear data have proven that the occurrence of cerebral microemboli may be related to clear neurologic events. However, in a first study using the transcranial Doppler technique (TCD), it could be demonstrated, that during CAS with a distal balloon neuroprotection (Percusurge Guard Wire™) the counts of microembolic signals (MES) were significantly reduced in comparison to CAS performed without protection.

In a second recent study of our group, the effectivity of a filter device versus proximal endovascular clamping was tested using the TCD as detector of MES during CAS.

The use of the Mo.Ma system significantly reduced MES in comparison to the filter used (EPI Filter Wire EX) not only during wiring of the stenosis, but also and predominantly during stent deployment and postdilatation.

These findings could suggest that filters are not completely able to prevent emboli, either because of insufficient vessel wall alignment or because a considerable amount of debris is too small

(< 100 μm) to be completely captured by the currently available systems.

The TCD findings, however, are not correlated with the clinical outcome. This fact indicates that during CAS clinically silent embolizations occur. First clinical studies using the very sensitive diffusion-weighted magnetic resonance imaging (DW-MRI) are confirming that cerebral lesions were observed in 30% of CAS performed without neuroprotection.

Utilizing filters, asymptomatic lesions were still seen in 23% of the cases. Finally, preliminary results in our institution indicate that proximal endovascular clamping seems not to completely prevent asymptomatic microembolic events (10–15%).

More extensive, controlled, multicenter studies are mandatory to better understand the dynamic mechanisms related to CAS and the value of the different neuroprotection techniques.

Unquestionable should be the fact that protection devices, in general, are safe and effective capturing particulate debris in 60–80% of the cases.

Filter devices seem to have the advantage of an easy handling, however, the disadvantages of the actual concepts are not trivial.

In particular, the flexibility and trackability of the systems have to be improved. It will remain impossible to control the adaptation to the vessel wall and, consequently, the efficacy of the filter during the intervention. Therefore,

the need for models simulating different anatomic situations in vitro is evident to demonstrate a priori the validity of the different devices.

Using filters, the clinical relevance of the underestimated occurrence of distal spasms – not yet evaluated in recent studies – has to be reconsidered. In this context an improvement of the stabilization of the filter position during the procedure should be discussed and realized.

Using proximal protection devices with endovascular clamping, it is important to consider the need for a 9-F sheath. This fact seems not to be correlated to a higher incidence of local complication (3.2% in the Mo.Ma™ registry, without surgical repair, using 10-F).

A further limitation of endovascular clamping is that a significant disease of the ECA may preclude the use of the system *(Figure 7)*.

In case of a contralateral occlusion of the ICA, an increased possibility of intolerance to flow blockage has to be taken into account selecting the patient. In such cases an intermittent deblockage of the antegrade flow may allow a successful step-by-step procedure.

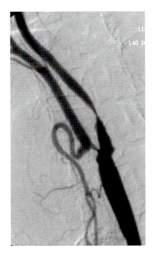

FIGURE 7. *Due to the ECA stenosis the use of a Mo.Ma system is not recommended.*

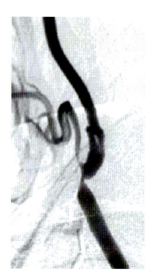
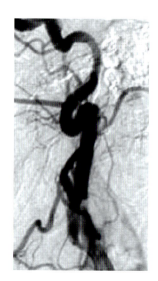
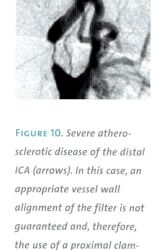

Figure 8. *Restenosis of the carotid bifurcation after surgery, where a proximal clamping device is not appropriate.*

Figure 9. *Severe kinking of the ICA distal to the stenosis where the use of a filter device is not reasonable.*

Figure 10. *Severe atherosclerotic disease of the distal ICA (arrows). In this case, an appropriate vessel wall alignment of the filter is not guaranteed and, therefore, the use of a proximal clamping device is recommended.*

The rare case of a bifurcational stenosis or lesion of the distal CCA is also not appropriate for the use of the proximal clamping device *(Figure 8)*.

On the other hand, in case of a severe kinking of the ICA distal to the stenosis *(Figure 9)* or in case of an apparently calcified distal ICA *(Figure 10)* the use of a filter device is not recommended or even not possible.

Stent Selection

In the initial phase of carotid stenting balloon-premounted stents have been used. Nowadays, practically only self-expandable stents are in use. There are no valuable scientific data demonstrating the superiority of any type of self-expandable stent independently of the anatomy, the structure or supposed composition of the obstructing lesion on the one hand as well as the design and the metal used on the other hand.

The first dedicated stent for the ICA was the Carotid Wallstent (Boston Scientific, Natick, MA, USA). This stent has been widely implanted around the world. The mesh design of this stainless-steel stent provides high plaque coverage. A constant radial force prevents collapsing of the plaque and allows embedding of the stent in the vessel wall. It adapts to the changing diameter of the vessel across the bifurcation very well.

A potential disadvantage of the Wallstent is its tendency to straighten the vessel imposing relevant changes of the original anatomy. An ulterior problem is related to the marked foreshortening (up to 30%) according to the diameter of the vessel so that an exact placement may be difficult.

The Carotid Wallstent comes in a diameter of 6–10 mm and has a nominal length of 30–50 mm. It is a rapid exchange system compatible with a 0.014" wire. The outer diameter of the delivery system is 5 or 5.9 F.

An alternative to the stainless-steel Wallstent are the newer generation of self-expanding stents, the nitinol stents: RX Acculink (Guidant, Indianapolis, IN, USA), Precise (Cordis, Miami Lakes, FL, USA), Exponent (Medtronic, Minneapolis, MN, USA), Xact Carotid Stent (Abbott, Abbott Place, IL, USA), Sinus-Carotid, (Optimed, Ettlingen, Germany), Conformexx (Nard, Murray Hill, NJ, USA), Zilver Stent (Cook, Bloomington, IN, USA) Protégé GPS (ev3, Plymouth, MN, USA). Different types with either an open-cell or closed-cell design, straight or tapered forms as well as different diameters and length of the stents are available. The NexStent (Boston Scientific Corp., Natick, MA, USA), a closed-cell nitinol stent with a 5-F delivery system, has a unique design and is formed like a carpet which allows the use of one stent size for vessels with a diameter of 4–10 mm.

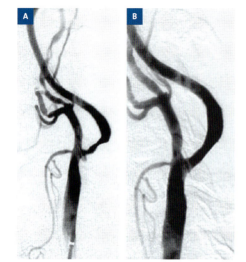

FIGURES 11A AND 11B.
a) Angulated origin of the ICA.
b) Result after implantation of a nitinol stent.

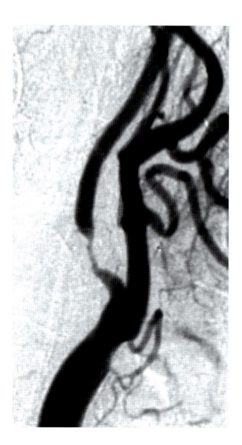

FIGURE 12.
Stenosis of the ICA appropriate for the use of a tapered stent.

Stent Deployment

The stent selection is extremely operator-dependent, often without any proven rationale.

In case of tortous ICA or angulated origin *(Figures 11a and b)* of the ICA, we tend to use nitinol stents with an open-cell structure. In case of an evident discrepancy between the diameter of the ICA and the CCA or distal and proximal ICA *(Figure 12)*, we normally implant tapered stents.

The recommendation to use stents with a diameter 1–2 mm larger than the widest vessel diameter to be covered is not based on scientific data. Nevertheless, the most commonly used stents are those with a diameter of 6–8 mm, if the stent is placed only in the ICA, or of 8–10 mm, if the stent is deployed over the bifurcation. Although the ICA is 2–3 mm smaller than the CCA, oversizing the stent does not cause any acute or late problems.

We tend to routinely deploy the stent over the bifurcation also in case of absence of a clear involvement of the bifurcation or of the CCA in the obstructive process.

Overstenting the ECA is safe and does rarely cause an occlusion.

Postdilatation

We strongly recommend to avoid any type of overstretching during the postdilatation process that is necessary in the majority of the cases particularly after primary stenting.

The balloon diameter should be equal to the diameter of the ICA distal of the stent. Usually, we use sizes between 4.0 and 5.5 mm.

Larger balloons might squeeze the atherosclerotic material through the stent mesh. For a successful angioplasty a rest stenosis of 20% is acceptable.

We have to keep in mind that the stent, after deployment, will try to reach the nominal diameter ulteriorly expanding over time.

If there are segments of contrast-filled ulcerations external to the stent, they do not have to be obliterated. Post-stent dilatation of the stent segment placed in the CCA is not necessary and not recommended.

If the ECA becomes significantly stenosed or occluded after postdilatation of the stent, this vessel can be approached through the stent mesh and reopened. Usually, however, there is no need to do this.

Periprocedural Therapy

At least 3 days before the intervention all patients have to receive acetylsalicylic acid (ASS) 100 mg and clopidogrel 75 mg daily. If impossible, ASS 500 mg intravenously and clopidogrel 300 mg per os have to be administered 1h before the intervention.

In addition, heparin, usually 5,000–10,000 IU, is given to obtain an activated clotting time (ACT) of 200–250 s.

In our institution, atropine 1 mg is given i.v. routinely 1–2 min before the first dilatation or primary stenting.

We recommend to have a dopamine infusion ready to start, because the baroreceptor reaction particularly in elderly hypertonic patients may be severe provoking a frequency-independent negative hemodynamic reaction with hypotension lasting sometimes for hours.

Postinterventionally, we routinely continue the combination of ASS and clopidogrel for at least 4 weeks. Thereafter, ASS 100 mg is given for an undetermined period.

Complications

Embolic Complications

The use of embolic protection systems has substantially reduced the risk of intraprocedural stroke. Nevertheless, the probability of an acute minor neurologic deficit during the procedure is still in a range of 2.0–4.0%. During the procedure, it is nearly impossible in the majority of the cases to differentiate between an embolic and an ischemic complication. Whenever possible, the procedure should not be interrupted but concluded as rapidly as possible.

Adjunctive heparin (2,000–3,000 IU) should be administered if the ACT is < 300 s.

After conclusion of the procedure and reassessment of the patient, an intracranial angiography should be considered only in case of a clearly persistent deficit.

Comparing to the preprocedural intracranial angiography, vessel embolization may be detected. If there is no sign of embolism, a CT scan should be performed.

If there is no evidence of occlusion of the middle or anterior cerebral artery or one of their major branches, the probability of a full recovery is very high. Only if the M1 or M2 segment of the middle cerebral artery remains occluded a mechanical intervention should be planed.

In a first step, the passage of an hydrophilic wire through the obstruction may be sufficient to restore flow. In some cases, a gentle dilatation with a small coronary balloon (1.5 or 2.0 mm) may solve the problem.

Normally, the embolic material is not thrombotic in nature but represents a sclerotic fragment embolized during the procedure so that an adjunctive lytic therapy is of limited value and may provoke a hemorrhagic complication.

Carotid Artery Spasm

In contrast to the CCA, the ICA tends to manifest an immediate reaction to manipulation with wires and other devices. The spasms may occur in multiple positions and simulate a functional occlusion of the distal ICA.

Such reactions are particularly undesirable using distal filters, because in such cases a differentiation between a debris-induced flow blockage and spasm is not possible. In such cases we try to conclude the intervention as soon as possible after injection of 0.1–0.2 mg of nitroglycerin.

Normally, spasms vanish spontaneously after several minutes when the devices are removed. The intervention should not be considered concluded before the phenomenon is solved or at least improved. In dependence on the hemodynamic situation, nitroglycerin can be repeatedly administered through the sheath. Particularly in patients with a contralateral occlusion, severe spasm may induce severe neurologic symptoms; surprisingly enough this type of temporary flow blockage is usually well tolerated without detectable symptoms.

Spasms of the ECA are rare and do not require treatment.

Poststenting Hypotension

Hypotension after conclusion of the procedure is not uncommon. Therefore, monitoring of the blood pressure should be mantained in all patients. In case of a contralateral occlusion or an intracranial stenosis, the systolic blood pressure should be maintained at a level of 120–140 mmHg or even higher.

Usually, hypotension is mediated by the persisting stretch of the baroreceptors induced by the self-expanding stent. Occasionally, hypotension can persist for days and may be a problem in the management of hypertensive patients. Other causes of hypotension such as retroperitoneal bleeding should be excluded.

Hyperfusion Syndrome

Cerebral hemorrhage as a consequence of increased blood flow after stenting is a rare complication (< 0.5%). Predictive factors may be an excessive anticoagulation in combination with uncontrolled hypertension. Patients with a recent ischemic event within the preceding 3 weeks may also tend to show this complication.

The symptoms are often diffuse, varying extremely on intensity. A typical symptom is the development of unconsciousness, sometimes preceded with severe headache. If there is no support of an ischemic event, anticoagulation should be reversed with protamine and a CT scan should be performed immediately.

It is important to know that symptoms of a hyperperfusion syndrom are seldom within the first hours after intervention.

External Carotid Artery Occlusions

An occlusion of the ECA is rarely caused by stenting of the ICA. Usually, it produces no symptoms due to good collaterals from the contralateral ECA.

After CAS, patients very rarely complain of pain when masticating, especially if the ECA is jailed.

In some patients the ECA can partially supply the brain through collaterals via the ophthalmic artery and pial collateral branches. In those patients it can be considered to maintain the patency of the ECA. With coronary balloon techniques the vessel can be reached through the mesh of the stent. It has not to be opened completely as long as sufficient blood flow is provided.

Carotid Dissection

Carotid dissection is often associated with very tortuous and calcified lesions. It might be caused maneuvering a distal protection device through the lesion or by the delivery system of self-expanding stents particularly in distal lesions. During positioning of the guiding sheath, a dissection of the CCA may occur. To avoid flow disruption, it might be necessary to deliver an ulterior stent in the area of dissection.

Carotid Perforation

This extremely rare complication might be the consequence of an oversizing of the postdilatation balloon. If encountered, prolonged balloon inflation may seal it. Covered stents can be used to solve the problem.

Clinical Results

Large case series have been reported from cardiology, interventional radiology, vascular surgery and neuroradiology centers *(Table 1)*. The results have suggested that CAS can be accomplished safely in a relatively large group of patients *(Figure 13)*.

The results of CAS have to be compared to CEA which is still the gold standard in treating carotid stenoses in symptomatic and asymptomatic patients *(Table 1)*.

In the cohorts analyzed in the relevant studies (NASCET;ECST;ACAS and ACST) the indications for CEA were relatively well defined:

- (1.) **Symptomatic patients < 80 years, with > 50% carotid stenosis, if the surgical risk for stroke and death is < 6–7%.**
- (2.) **Asymptomatic patients < 80 years, with > 60% carotid stenosis, if the surgical risk for stroke and death is < 3%.**

Similar, clear definitions for CAS indications are not available at the moment. In fact in the majority of the single- and multicenter registries the patients selected for CAS showed a higher risk stratification.

In particular, the indication has been extended to patients > 80 years of age.

Nevertheless, based on a review of the results of the ARCHER I–III registries

TABLE 1.

Study	Treatment	Patients	Death/stroke (%)
NASCET	CEA[1]	1,087	6.7
ACAS	CEA	825	2.3
VACS	CEA	195	4.4
CAVATAS	CEA	240	10.4
	CAS[2]	246	10.2
Roubin et al.	CAS	528	7.1
Wholey et al.	CAS	4,749	5.9
SAPPHIRE	CEA	151	6.6
	Protected CAS	156	4.5
ARCHeR	Protected CAS	437	6.6
Mo.Ma	Protected CAS	157	5.7
Priamus (Mo.Ma)	Protected CAS	416	4.5

[1] CEA : carotid endarterectomy   [2] CAS: carotid artery stenting

TABLE 1. Death and stroke rate of relevant CEA- and CAS-studies.

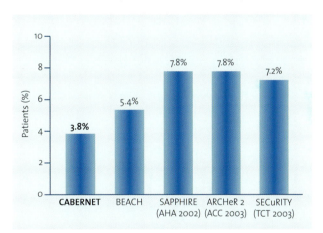

FIGURE 13. 30-Day Composite Endpoint in US Carotid Stenting Registries

the Acculink Carotid Stent plus ACCUNET™ Embolic Protection Device (Guidant) was the first system which received the FDA approval on August 31, 2004.

The devices have been released for use in patients who have had symptoms of a stroke or who have a carotid artery blockage of at least 80%, and who are not good candidates for endarterectomy.

This is a very weak definition permitting a wide range of possible interpretations.

The recently published data of the SAPPHIRE study will probably permit to transform the preliminary approval of the system into a final clearance for its use in high-risk patients.

The SAPPHIRE study is the first randomized study comparing CEA with protected CAS in which it could be demonstrated that CAS is not inferior to endarterectomy. The primary endpoint, death, stroke or myocardial infarction at 30 days plus ipsilateral stroke or death from neurologic causes within 31 days and 1 year, occurred in 20.1% after CEA and 12.2% after stenting (p = 0.05).

The results of these studies and of other registries may dramatically change the scenario for the treatment of carotid obstructive disease.

It is important to stress the fact that after CAS the restenosis rate is remarkably low, compared to other vascular interventions. Several authors reviewing larger series report a rate between 2.3% and 5%. Most restenoses occur within 6–12 months after the intervention. In our own experience, the incidence of restenoses in the last 2 years is lower.

Summary

A dramatic improvement of dedicated tools for CAS has been observed during the last few years.

Nevertheless, the CAS procedure remains challenging and requires an absolutely perfect and complete armamentarium permitting the selection of the dedicated optimal material for every single patient.

However, the refinements of the systems cannot replace the mandatory necessity of an adequate and controlled training of each interventionalist starting the CAS program.

References

1. Adami CA, Scuro A, Spinamano L. Use of the parodi anti-embolism system in carotid stenting: Italian trial results. J Endovasc Ther 2002;9:147–54.
2. Al-Mubarak N, Colombo A, Gaines PA. Multicenter evaluation of carotid artery stenting with a filter protection system. J Am Coll Cardiol 2002;6:841–6.
3. Al-Mubarak N, Roubin GS, Vitek JJ. Effect of the distal-balloon protection system on microembolization during carotid stenting. Circulation 2001;104:1999–2002.
4. Antonius Carotid Endarterectomy, Angioplasty, and Stenting Study Group. Transcranial Doppler monitoring in angioplasty and stenting of the carotid bifurcation. J Endovasc Ther 2003;10:702–10.
5. Birkmeyer JD, Stukel TA, Siewers AE. Surgeon volume and operative mortality in the United States. N Engl J Med 2003;349:2117–27.
6. Castriota F, Cremosesi A, Manetti R. Impact of cerebral protection devices on early outcome of carotid stenting. J Endovasc Ther 2002;9:786–92.
7. Cremonesi A, Manetti R, Setacci F. Protected carotid stenting: clinical advantages and complications of embolic protection devices in 442 consecutive patients. Stroke 2003;34:1936–41.
8. Diederich KW, Scheinert D, Schmidt A. First clinical experiences with an endovascular clamping system for neuroprotection during carotid stenting. Eur J Vasc Endovasc Surg 2004;28,629–33.
9. Endarterectomy for asymptomatic carotid artery stenosis. Executive Committee for the Asymptomatic Carotid Atherosclerosis Study. JAMA 1995;273:1421–8.
10. Endovascular versus surgical treatment in patients with carotid stenosis in the Carotid and Vertebral Artery Transluminal Angioplasty Study (CAVATAS): a randomized trial. Lancet 2001;357:1729–37.
11. European Carotid Surgery Trialists' Collaborative Group. MRC European Carotid Surgery Trial: interim results for symptomatic patients with servere (70–99%) or with mild (0–29%) carotid stenosis. Lancet 1991;337:1235–43.
12. Gray WA, et al. A cardiologist in the carotids. J Am Coll Cardiol 2004;43:1602–5.
13. Henry M, Amor M, Henry I. Carotid stenting with cerebral protection: first clinical experience using the percusurge guardwire system. J Endovasc Surg 1999;6:321–31.
14. Hertzer NR, et al. Results of carotid endarterectomy: the gold standard for carotid repair. Semin Vasc Surg 2000;13:95–102.
15. Jaeger HJ, Mathias KD, Hauth E. Cerebral ischemia detected with diffusion-weighted MR imaging after stent implantation in the carotid artery. AJNR Am J Neuroradiol 2002;23:200–7.
16. MCR Asymptomatic Carotid Surgery Trial (ACST) Collaborative Group. Prevention of disabling and fatal strokes by successful carotid endarterectomy in patients without recent neurological symptoms: randomized controlled trial. Lancet 2004;363:.
17. North American Symptomatic Carotid Endarterectomy Trial Collaborators. Beneficial effect of carotid endarterectomy in symptomatic patients with high-grade stenosis. N Engl J Med 1991;325:445–53.
18. Ohki T, Roubin GS, Veith FJ. Efficacy of a filter device in the prevention of embolic events during carotid angioplasty and stenting: an ex vivo analysis. J Vasc Surg. 1999;30:1034–44.
19. Ouriel K, Hertzer NR, Beven EG. Preprocedural risk stratification: identifying an appropriate population for carotid stenting. J Vasc Surg 2001;33:728–32.
20. Reimers B, Corvaja N, Moshiri S. Cerebral protection with filter devices during carotid artery stenting. Circulation 2001;104:12–15.
21. Reimers B, Schlüter M, Castriota F. Routine use of cerebral protection during carotid artery stenting: results of a multicenter registry of 753 patients. Am J Med 2004;116:217–22.
22. Reimers B, Sievert H, Schuler GC. Proximal endovascular flow blockage for cerebral protection during carotid artery stenting: results from a prospective multicenter registry. J Endovasc Ther 2005;12:156–65.
23. Roubin GS, New G, Iyer SS. Immediate and late clinical outcomes of carotid artery stenting in patients with symptomatic and asymptomatic carotid artery stenosis: a 5-year prospective analysis. Circulation 2001;103:532–7.
24. Schlüter M, Tübler T, Mathey DG. Feasibility and efficacy of balloon-based neuroprotection during carotid artery stenting in a single-center setting. J Am Coll Cardiol 2002;40:890–95.
25. Schmidt A, Diederich KW, Scheinert S, Bräunlich S, Olenburger T, Biamino G, Schuler G, Scheinert D. Effect of two different neuroprotection systems on microembolization during carotid artery stenting. J Am Coll Cardiol 2004;16:1966-9.
26. Sievert H, Rabe K, Biamino G. Technique and results of carotid stenting. PCR 2004;335.
27. Wholey MH, Wholey M, Mathias K. Global experience in cervical carotid artery stent placement. Cathet Cardiovasc Interv 2000;50:160–7.
28. Yadav JS, Roubin GS, Iyer S. Elective stenting of the extracranial carotid arteries. Circulation 1997;95:376–81.
29. Yadav JS, Wholey MH, Kuntz RE. Protected carotid-artery stenting versus endarterectomy in high-risk patients. N Engl J Med 2004;351:1493–501.
30. Zahn R, Mark B, Niedermaier N. Embolic protection devices for carotid artery stenting: better results than stenting without protection? Eur Heart J 2004;25:1550–8.

Index

A

AAA-rupture 138
AAA-symptoms 126
abdominal aortic aneurysm (AAA) 125
activated clotting time 167
AL 1 guide 149
angiography, intracranial 150, 168
angiography, pelvic arteries 29
Ankle-Brachial Index (ABI) 11
antegrade access 47, 77
aortic arch 145
aortic balloon catheter 113
aortic dissection 118-122
    classification 118
    endovascular procedure 120
    incidence 118
    mortality 118
aortic stent 38
aortoiliac bifurcation
    kissing balloon technique 37
    reconstruction 37

B

balloon angioplasty, tibial arteries 80, 88
balloon catheter, low-profile 80, 88
bovine arch 149
brachial approach 103, 129, 147
buddy wires 157
bypass surgery, CLI 75

C

carotid artery spasm 168
carotid artery stenting 143
    activated clotting time 167
    angiography, intracranial 150, 168
    aortic arch 146
    bovine arch 149
    brachial approach 147
    complications 168–170
        carotid dissection 170
        carotid perforation 170
        carotid spasm 168
        embolic 168
        hyperperfusion syndrome 170
        hypotension 169
        ischemic 168
    coronary approach 149
    diagnostic catheter 145
    embolic protection devices 153
        distal occlusion balloon 153
        endovascular clamping 158
        filter 156
        Mo.Ma system 159
        Parodi AES 158
    guiding catheter 150
    nitroglycerin 169
    post stenting hypotension 169
    postdilatation 167

carotid artery stenting (cont.)
    predilatation 152
    pull and push technique 146
    restenosis rate 172
    sheath 150
    stents 165
    telescoping technique 148
    vascular access 145
catheter
    Bernstein 145
    Diver 65, 77
    Hook 46
    Judgkins 46
    Mani 147
    Omni Selective 46
    Right Judkins 146
    Shepherd´s Hook 46
    Sidewinder 145, 147
    Simmons 147
    vertebralis 145
    Vitek 145, 147
    Cobra 46
cerebral micro emboli 162
contrast-enhenced spiral CT 112
critical limb ischemia (CLI) 71
    bypass surgery 75
    patency rates 75
    physical examination 74
    prognosis 71
crossover access 34, 46, 76
crossover sheath 34, 47
crossover, step-by-step 34
cutting balloon 53, 63

D

distal filter 153
distal landing zone 127
distal occlusion balloon 153
dopamine 167
Doppler waveform 14
DREAM trial 125, 134
drug-eluting stents 89
duplex sonography,
color-coded 13, 73
    pelvic arteries 13
    infrapopliteal arteries 16, 73
    infrageniculate arteries 16
    internal carotid artery 17
    supraaortic arteries 17, 144
    subclavian artery 20
    renal artery 22, 97
    femoral arteries 14, 46
Dutch Iliac Stent Trial 27

E

embolic neurological event 153
endografting, complications 134
endoleak 115, 127, 134, 135
endoprosthesis 113
    oversizing of - 112
endotension 134
endovascular aneurysm repair
(EVAR) 111
    abdominal aorta 125
        complications 135
            AAA rupture 138
            endoleak 127, 135–137
            graft occlusion 138
            migration 136
            modular component
            separation 134, 137
        endovascular procedure 129
        follow-up 131
        hypogastric artery 127
        patient selection 126
        post dilatation 131
        postinterventional
        treatment 131
        stent graft devices 128
        suprarenal fixation 130
    thoracic aorta 111
        aortic dissection 118
        aortic rupture 117
        endoprosthesis sizing 112
        endovascular procedure 112, 120
        guide wire 113
        paraplegia 115
        postdilatation 120
        postinterventional
        treatment 113
        subclavian artery 113
        type 1 endoleak 115
EUROSTAR registry 139
EVAR-1 trial 125, 134
excimer laser 54, 82
    debulking technique 83
    laser physics 54
    step-by-step technique 54, 82

F

femoropopliteal artery 46
    access techniques 46
    acute occlusion 64
    balloon angioplasty 52
    diagnostic work-up 46
    embolisation 68
    excimer laser 54
    guide wires 49
    guiding catheters 50
    occlusions, acute and
    subacute 64
    perforation 67
    pioneer catheter 50
    stenting 56
        indications 60
        nitinol stent 58–59
        stent fracture 63
        Wallstent 57
    subintimal recanalisation 49
    Terumo wire 49
    total occlusion 49
    transpopliteal technique 48
fibromuscular dysplasia 105
filter systems 156
    premounted 158
focal iliac artery stenosis 27
Fontaine staging 10

G

guide wire 77
    carotid arteries 158, 159
    femoral arteries 49
    infrapopliteal arteries 77
    pelvic arteries 36
    renal arteries 101
    ultrastiff 113

H

hockey stick 151
hyperperfusion syndrome 170
hypogastric artery 127

I

iliac artery occlusions, chronic 36
iliac artery stenosis 39
iliac artery interventions 27-43
    aortoiliac bifurcation 37
    approach 32
        crossover 34
        retrograde 32
        transbrachial 35
    chronic occlusion 36
    balloon expandable stents 30
    patency rates 39-41
    postinterventional treatment 38
    stents 30, 31
    TASC working group 27, 28
IMA catheter 46

infrapopliteal 71-93
    access methods 76-77
    balloon-dilatation 80
    bypass Surgery 75
    color-coded duplex sonography 73
    complications 85
    critical limb ischemia 71
        differential diagnosis 74
        ischemic rest pain 73
        nonhealing ulceration 73
        physical examination 74
        neuropathy 74
    drug-eluting stents 89
    guide wire 77
    laser recanalization 82, 90-92
    low-profile balloons 80
    patency 75, 88
    postprocedural treatment 86
    stents 84, 88
    success rate 76, 88
    support-catheter 77
infrarenal aorta, obstruction 41
INSTEAD trial 122
internal carotid artery (ICA) 155–157
intermittend claudication 73
ischemic rest pain 73

K

kissing balloon technique 37, 38

L

LACI trial 90
limb salvage 76
low-profile balloon catheter 80, 88

M

medial calcification 11
middle cerebral artery 168
Mo.Ma European Registry 160
Mo.Ma neuroprotection device 159
MR angiography 96, 144

N

neurologic examination 152

O

occlusions, acute and subacute 64
ostial lesions 31, 38, 105
oversizing of endoprosthesis 112

P

paraplegia 115, 122
patency rates 39
    carotid arteries 172
    femoral arteries 53, 57, 58
    infrapopliteal arteries 75, 88, 89
    pelvic arteries 39
    pelvic artery interventions
        see iliac artery interventions
pelvic arteries, angiography 29
peripheral neuropathy 74
postdilatation 120, 131, 167
Priamus registry 160
proximal endovascular clamping 153
proximal entry site 119
proximal entry tear 120
proximal fixation zone 127
proximal neck 112
pseudoclaudication 12
pulse curve recording 11

R

radial access 145
remodeling of aorta 119
renal artery 22, 95
   angiographic evaluation 100
   angioplasty 98
      indications 98
      techniques 101
   arterial hypertension 98
   coaxial technique 102
   guide wire technique 101
   guiding-catheter technique 103
   low profile stents 107
   MR angiography 96
   noninvasive testing 96
   renal insufficiency 99
   rupture 108
   screening 96
   stenting 105
   stents 107
renal double curve 103
renal insufficiency 99
Resistive Index (RI) 23, 99
retrograde iliac approach 32
rupture of aortic type B dissection 116
rupture of preexisting atherosclerotic thoracic aneurysm 116
Rutherford classification 10

S

SAPPHIRE study 172
self-expanding stents 30
sirolimus-eluting balloon-expandable stents 89
spasm 85, 157
   carotid artery 168
   distal 163
spiral computed tomography 97
stent 56
   abdominal stent grafts 128
   aortic 38
   balloon-expandable 30, 84
   carotid 165
   drug-eluting 89
   femoral 57
   iliac 30
   infrapopliteal 88
   in-stent restenosis 62
   nitinol stent 31, 57, 59, 61, 165
   renal 107
   self expanding 30, 84, 165
   tibial 73, 88
   Wallstent 30, 56, 57, 165
step-by-step technique 82
subclavian artery 113
subclavian steal phenomenon 20
support catheter 65, 77
suprarenal fixation 130
surgical access, extraperitoneal 129

T

telescoping technique 148
thoracic aortic aneurysm 111
   access vessel 113
   clinical manifestation 111
   mortality rates 111
   natural history 111
   noninvasive workup 111
   postinterventional treatment 113
   surgical repair 111
thrombectomy, mechanical 64
thrombolysis 66
thrombus, local 85
tibial arteries, stenting 73, 88
TransAtlantic Inter-Society Consensus (TASC) Working Group 27, 53
transbrachial access 35, 145
transcranial Doppler technique (TCD) 162
transesophageal echocardiography 119
transpopliteal technique 48
treadmill testing 12

V

V18-control-wire 49

W

weighted magnetic resonance imaging (DW-MR) 163

Dierk Scheinert, MD

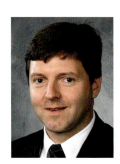

After medical study at the Humboldt University of Berlin, he began his postgraduate training in internal medicine at the University Hospital Charité – Campus Virchow Klinikum. Early on he became involved with peripheral interventional work at the Department of Clinical and Interventional Angiology of the Virchow Klinikum, which since then has remained the primary focus of his clinical and scientific work. After training in cardiology at the University Hospital Erlangen-Nuremberg from 1999 till 2001, Dr. Scheinert moved to the University of Leipzig – Heart Center to build up the peripheral interventional program together with Professor Biamino and Dr. Schmidt. Since 2003 he is the Director of the Department of Clinical and Interventional Angiology at the Heart Center Leipzig and since 2005 Head of the Department of Internal Medicine I – Angiology and Cardiology at the Park Hospital Leipzig.

Dr. Scheinert's main clinical and scientific interest is the advancement of interventional techniques for complex peripheral obstructions, which was also the topic of his habilitation in internal medicine.

Andrej Schmidt, MD

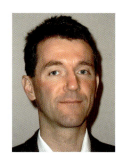

After medical study at the Free University Berlin, he began his postgraduate training in internal medicine at the Carl Gustav Carus Hospital of the Technical University of Dresden. It was there that he started his activity as an angiologist with specialization in duplex ultrasound and conservative treatment of PAOD in 1995. After moving to the University of Erlangen-Nuremberg in 1998, he became involved in endovascular treatment of PAOD and completed his specialization in internal medicine, cardiology and angiology. Together with Dr. Scheinert, he moved to the University of Leipzig – Heart Center in 2001, where since then he has worked mainly as an interventionalist.

Dr. Schmidt's main clinical and scientific interest is the interventional treatment of carotid disease and patients with critical limb ischemia.

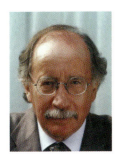

Giancarlo Biamino, MD

Having studied medicine at the Free University of Berlin, he started his career as a medical assistant in the Institute of Physiology of the Medical Clinic and Policlinic at Klinikum Steglitz of the Free University of Berlin. In 1969 he became a guest assistant at the Physiological Institute of the University of Göteborg. Habilitation in "Physiology and Clinical Physiology" (1970) and "Internal Medicine" (1975) at the Free University of Berlin. In 1979 nomination to full professor in medicine at the Free University of Berlin. In 1984 he became guest professor at the Mid American Heart Institution in Kansas City.

Starting 1989, he headed the Cardiovascular Project on Laser Angioplasty at the Laser Medizin Zentrum Berlin. At the same time he became Head of the Department of Laser Angioplasty at the University Hospital Charité – Campus Virchow Klinikum, where he also chaired the Department of Clinical and Interventional Angiology, until he moved to Hamburg in 1998.

From 2002 to 2006 he directed the Department of Clinical and Interventional Angiology at the Heart Center Leipzig.

Since 2004 he is a consulting interventionalist at the Cardiovascular Center in Frankfurt/Main. In spring 2006 he has been nominated Chairman of the Gruppo Villa Maria Endovascular, Italy.

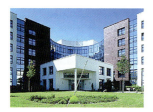

Heart Center Leipzig

The Department of Clinical and Interventional Angiology at the University of Leipzig – Heart Center and Park Hospital Leipzig started its work in 1998 and has since then experienced a constantly growing number of admitted patients. More than 2,000 peripheral interventions were performed during the year 2005, mostly in the femoro-popliteal, infrapopliteal and pelvic arteries. Beyond that, carotid interventions as well as stent graft implantations for endovascular repair of aortic pathologies represent important clinical and research fields of our department.

Recently, treatment of critical limb ischemia, especially the interventional treatment of pathologies of below-the-knee arteries, became one of the most important and rapidly growing fields of our clinical activity.

A main focus of our department is clinical research in the field of vascular disease. Moreover, we are strongly committed to clinical teaching programs with the aim of making interventional techniques more widely available. In that context, the angiologic working group is constantly invited to participate in national and international meetings and congresses by performing a high number of live cases (e.g., EURO PCR, TCT, ISET, All That Jazz, CCT). Recently, the Leipzig Interventional Course (LINC) was initiated, which already after this year's second edition turned out to be one of the most successful live courses in the field of peripheral vascular intervention *(www.leipzig-interventional-course.de)*.